SENIOR FITNESS
FOR PAIN RELIEF

A 4-WEEK WORKOUT PROGRAM DESIGNED TO
REDUCE PAIN, INCREASE YOUR MOBILITY AND
BOOST YOUR ENERGY

MARK SHAW

TABLE OF CONTENTS

A FREE GIFT TO ALL MY READERS!

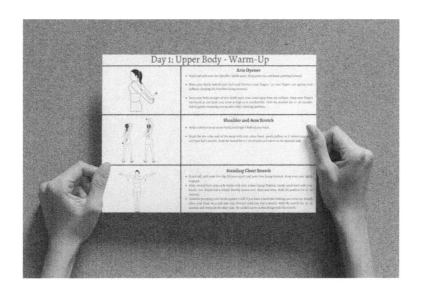

As a thank you, and to help you make the most of your new fitness routine, I would like to share a workout log recapping all the exercises and the stretches presented in the book. The log comes with illustrations and plenty of space to take notes. Hopefully it will serve you as a quick reference during your workout.

To download it, please scan the QR code below!

AUTHOR'S NOTE

Hello reader, thanks again for purchasing my book! I have an important message for you: there is no need to read this book from start to finish or sequentially. I did my best to make it as comprehensive as possible. As a result, some chapters may be irrelevant or unnecessary to certain readers. Please bear in mind that every chapter touches on a unique topic and can be read on its own or skipped altogether. Feel free to skip the chapters that don't interest you. Alternatively, you can read the book from start to finish for a deeper look at Senior Fitness. The choice is yours.

INTRODUCTION

And I said to my body, softly, 'I want to be your friend.' It took a long breath. And replied, 'I have been waiting my whole life for this. –Nayyirah Waheed

Maintaining an active lifestyle generally keeps us out of the hospital. It also improves our overall fitness and can help us manage health conditions and pain. Physical activity gives us the keys to steer the vehicle of our independence, all it asks for in return is some patience and dedication. I often think of my friend's grandmother, Chivonne, who, at 78 years old, still lives independently in her cottage. She maintains her health with daily walks, stretches, gardening, using resistance bands, and eating a balanced diet. It may sound like Chivonne has a lot on her plate, but in reality, her day probably looks very similar to yours. She'd regularly joke that she's in much better shape now than in her 30s! Looking at her now, one cannot tell that she experiences regular bouts of pain. Aunty Chivonne swears by her daily stretching regimen to manage pain, and for good reason. A daily stretch engages the parasympathetic nervous system, increases blood flow to the muscles, and releases endorphins–all of which combine to create that feel-good feeling after a good workout.

There is no need to resign yourself to a fate of slow decay that the loss of independence brings about. Perhaps you've taken the first steps, but feel discouraged and stuck with the results of previous fitness programs. The good news is that it is never too late to transform your life! That's precisely what this guide is for, to point you along the path of transformation. It is possible to enjoy your golden years with renewed vigor!

This fitness program was designed to meet you where you are, setting it apart from other programs. Typical fitness programs may not be designed for seniors or pain management and can accelerate too quickly. When fitness programs become too challenging, we quickly lose the habit because we are not seeing the results we are expecting when compared to the effort that's been exerted. This is why this guide takes a different approach. The focus here is to build on small gains to create a healthy and sustainable fitness habit. Each chapter will discuss different exercises and tips that are aimed at getting the maximum benefit from your fitness routine.

The beauty of exercise is that when you pass the first 28 days and start to experience the benefits, you'll be able to motivate yourself to keep the momentum going! It all starts with that first decision you take to reclaim your life. Hopefully, this is what we'll achieve together! This guide is filled with exercises and fitness programs designed to get you moving today still. Don't let pain and frailty stand in your way of living your best life.

CHAPTER 1

IT'S ABOUT QUALITY

Two hundred years ago, it was a milestone to live past 30 years of age. As the gears of progress and change turned, the average global life expectancy increased dramatically, more than doubling our lifespans when compared to our ancestors (Roser et al., 2013). Longer lifespans meant that we could do and experience so much more, but it comes with a price tag: An increased risk of pain, frailty, and other health complications. The question we are faced with now is: How do we increase the quality of life in our golden years? The answer is physical activity.

Physical activity has been identified as a protective factor against health conditions such as cardiovascular disease, diabetes, stroke, and some types of cancer (Langhammer et al., 2018). Physical activity can even delay the onset of dementia and make for a good pain management tool (Livingston et al., 2017). As benefit-filled as exercising in our golden years can be, some legitimate concerns prevent many of us from living our best lives.

Did you know that one of the first symptoms of an overly sedentary lifestyle manifests as joint pain? Pre-existing injuries, age-onset conditions, fear of injury, and a lack of mobility keep us trapped in the false security of immobility. Yes, our chances of falling are next to nothing if we spend most of our time on the couch, but this does our bodies no favors either. There is a fine line between allowing fear (whether it be of falling, pain, or other concerns) to control our actions and truly understanding a pre-existing condition. Whether you are embarking on a fitness journey for the first time or have been a longtime fitness junkie, one golden rule applies to everyone: Respect the limitations of your body. This essentially means that we:

- **_Face Fear:_** Acknowledge the possibility of falls and injury; thus we need to look for ways to prevent injury in our fitness regimen.

- **_Take It Slow:_** Be patient with your progress. Whether the goal is to reduce pain or to improve physique and mobility, we need to keep in mind that our bodies will grow stronger at their own rate. All we have to do is to be consistent in our fitness program. It is when we push ourselves beyond our limits that injuries occur.

- **_Get the Green Light:_** Always talk to your healthcare provider first before attempting or adjusting a fitness regimen. Your healthcare provider will be able to tell you which exercises are safe.

The key to respecting the golden rule is building our self-awareness and learning what we should avoid. I'll share a tip with you: Master form before dialing up the difficulty. There is an excellent reason why fitness professionals place so much emphasis on progressing with exercises slowly. It is to ensure that our form (posture, breathing, muscle clenching) is suited for the exercise. When we master form, exercising becomes a very safe activity that reduces the risk of injury and pain. Mastering form can be tricky at first, but it becomes easier as you gain experience and confidence in your new fitness regimen. Helping you master form and perform exercises safely for a pain-free life is one of the foundations on which this book is based.

THE BENEFITS OF FITNESS

Physical activity comes with a few neat perks, which we'll discuss below. From reducing pain to keeping us mobile, we'll take a closer look at how a little exercise can go a long way to enhancing the quality of life.

A Natural Painkiller

Ever wonder why opioids are sometimes prescribed for pain? It's because these substances trigger the release of endorphins in our bodies. Endorphins are our bodies' natural painkillers and can relieve stress, leaving us with that feel-good feeling. They are released by the hypothalamus and pituitary glands. Opioids (such as morphine, fentanyl, and tramadol) combat pain by mimicking the actions of endorphins by interacting with specific receptors in our bodies (*Endorphins: The brain's natural pain reliever*, 2021). The misuse and overuse of opioids can have dangerous and lasting consequences for our health and well-being, but what if I told you there is a non-prescription method to combat the pain? In fact, this method makes for a good complement to most pain management regimens. Yes, you already guessed it! Exercise is the answer. When we exercise at a moderate pace, our bodies release endorphins. That's why we feel so good and relaxed after a workout session.

Improved Sleep

Endorphins do more than combat pain. It helps us sleep better and can combat the frustrations of insomnia. Through exercise, we can rid ourselves of stress and anxiety, helping the brain enter "sleep mode" a lot easier. It also gets rid of excess energy in the body, helping us fall asleep easier without tossing and turning. The result is better quality sleep.

Reduces the Risk of Falling

No matter what age bracket we fall into, there is always a risk of falling and injuring ourselves. It's the tradeoff we bipeds have to live with. However, how we bounce back from a fall or injury is highly dependent on our level of physical fitness. Exercise helps to prevent falls because it makes our muscles strong and flexible, while improving balance and increasing the duration of how long we can be active (*Exercises to help prevent falls,* 2020). Incorporating simple, low-risk and low-energy movements into your daily routine is a good place to start strengthening our bodies if we've been sedentary for far too long.

Preserves Independence

People who exercise regularly can maintain their independence well into their golden years. This is why retired athletes often remain active, even at an advanced age. That's because regular exercise helps prevent the loss of muscle and bone mass. As we age, the nutrients that our bodies produce, consume, and maintain bone and muscle mass declines. This leads to our bones becoming brittle, making them prone to breakage. Our muscles can become stiff and weak, making it difficult to maintain an independent lifestyle. The good news is that regular physical activity and a healthy, balanced diet can help stave off the detrimental effects that weak bones and muscles have in store for us.

Keeps the Noggin Sharp

Cognitive decline is a scary reality many of us will face in our golden years, but there is a way to delay its onset. Keeping the mind active with puzzles and other mental drills is a great way to keep the mind sharp, but these efforts can be bolstered by the beneficial effects of exercise. That's because that post-workout endorphin rush helps to reset our brain's chemical balance, combating depression, anxiety, and stress in the process.

Can Delay Death From Other Causes

Physical activity helps us in three ways. Our muscles use the sugar available in our bloodstream to perform activities, thereby lowering our overall blood glucose levels. That's good news for those of us concerned about diabetes! Daily activity also lowers our blood pressure, reducing the risk of cardiovascular problems that are associated with it. Lastly, a daily burst of activity keeps the waistline in check, reducing our risk of contracting health complications linked to weight.

UNDERSTANDING EXERCISE

Now that we have a better understanding of the general positives that physical activity introduces into your lives, it is time to delve deeper and take a look at the types of exercise. Exercise can be divided into four main categories, namely:

- **Endurance:** Often referred to as aerobic exercises, these activities increase our breathing and heart rate. Endurance exercises are useful to improve our fitness levels and can keep your heart, lungs, and circulatory system functioning optimally. Don't worry! You don't need to bust out the colorful leg warmers that characterized Jane Fonda's workout days. A brisk walk, swimming, dancing, playing with the grandchildren, or climbing stairs all count as endurance exercises.

- **Strength:** Strength training keeps our muscles and posture strong and is a key ingredient to maintaining our independent lifestyles for longer. Strong, healthy muscles help to keep our posture erect, which improves our balance. It also reduces the risk of lower back pain that poor posture usually triggers. Strength training can be done with weights, resistance bands, or your body weight. To ensure your strength training is as safe as possible, always start with the lightest weight or weakest resistance band and work your way up from there. Never hold your breath during strength training exercises, either.

- **Balance:** Falls in older adults can have serious consequences, this is why every good fitness regimen should include exercises for balance. Many lower body exercises can improve our balance. When starting with balance exercises, be sure to practice them next to a sturdy surface (such as a table, chair, wall, or convenient counter) that you can use to steady yourself.

- **Flexibility:** A flexible body is a mobile one! As we grow older, it may become harder to look over our shoulders, or to bend down. Fortunately, there are many ways we can improve our flexibility, including adding simple sketches to our daily routine. Before starting your stretching routine, always make sure your muscles are warmed up. Stretches after endurance and strength exercises are recommended and will help the muscles relax after the workout. You should not experience any pain while stretching. If you experience pain or discomfort, stop immediately.

Tips and Common Questions

This section is a general compilation of tips to help you get started and achieve the best results possible on your fitness journey.

- Try to move as much as possible throughout the day. This small change can make quite a difference eventually.
- Aim to get at least 150 minutes of moderately intensive activity every week, or 75 minutes of vigorous activity (*Move More; Sit Less*, 2022).
- Dedicate at least two of your workout days to strength training.
- Include balance exercises in your workout.
- Ease into your fitness routine, increasing the intensity and duration slowly over time.
- Set realistic and attainable fitness goals for yourself.

Fill your exercise routine with movements that you enjoy. That way, it is much easier to commit to the routine and reap long-term benefits. By this point, you might have some burning fitness questions, to which you may find the answer in the section below.

What Is Considered an Aerobic Activity?

Aerobic activity is defined as any "activity that uses aerobic metabolism" (Iliades, MD, 2018). This means any activity that gets the blood flowing and our heart rate up counts as an aerobic activity. Playing ball with the grandchildren, walking in the park, biking, and dancing count as aerobic activities. Aerobic exercises can be easy and fun to work into our days.

What Is Workout Intensity?

'Intensity' refers to how hard we are working while exercising. Your fitness level will determine the intensity level. Keep in mind that everyone starts as a novice, so always increase the intensity of a workout in small increments.

What's the Difference Between "Moderate" and "Vigorous" Aerobic Exercise?

Given our previous definition of aerobic activity, we only need to ask ourselves which activities we find hard to breathe and keep up with. You are pushing yourself, but you are still able to talk with ease. That is moderate intensity. Vigorous intensity is only a little more hurried.

What Qualifies as Balance Activities?

Yoga and tai chi are known to improve our balance, but they might not appeal to everyone. Other exercises can easily be slipped into our daily routine, such as:

- Standing on one leg.
- Mimicking a tightrope walk (placing your heel directly in front of your toes).
- Sitting and rising from chairs without the use of your hands.
- Alternate lifting your knees to the chest as you walk.

Over time, as your balance improves, you'll find that you'll be able to hold the position for longer, add movement to the pose, or even let go of the support. It is recommended to do balance exercises at least twice a week, but they can be done daily (Watson, 2020).

Are Fitness Goals Important?

Fitness goals are wonderful tools. They hold us accountable and motivate us to make lasting changes to our lifestyles. However, the goals we decide on need to be realistic to be effective. Set smaller, manageable fitness targets that will help you achieve the goal.

How Does Inactivity Impact Health?

Sedentary lifestyles impact the whole body, increasing the risk of disease and doubling our chances of developing cardiovascular disease (*Physical inactivity a leading cause of disease and disability, warns WHO*, 2002). Inactivity is also linked to physical disability in older adults. That's because our muscles atrophy as we grow older, leaving our bodies ill-prepared for the demands of a modern lifestyle. However, our bodies are amazing in their adaptive capabilities, and even small, regular bouts of activity will pave the way for the health benefits mentioned earlier.

Is Exercise Safe for the Frail?

Yes, but talk to your healthcare provider first! Frailty is generally associated with muscle weakness, slow walking speed, fatigue, reduced activity, and unintentional weight loss. We usually become frail when experiencing chronic health challenges and problems related to aging. Regular physical activity can preserve or improve the functional status of our bodies, while conditioning muscles (Angulo et al., 2020). This makes exercise one of the best tools at our disposal to counter frailty and frailty-related impairment in our golden years.

Can I Exercise If I've Had a Hip Fracture?

Most older adults who experience a hip fracture also become frail (Sherrington et al., 2011). This does not have to be the case, however. Many people have found that gradual exercise programs can improve the outcomes of a hip fracture, allowing them to regain and maintain a good measure of independence.

Is It a Good Idea to Exercise With Osteoarthritis?

Absolutely! Exercise protects us from the damage that chronic inflammation can cause (Exercise: Rx for overcoming osteoarthritis, 2019). Moving around may be the last thing we'd feel like doing when our joints are achy and stiff, but physical activity can help to ease pain through the release of endorphins. It is best to talk to your healthcare provider for guidance on suitable activities.

How Does Physical Activity Influence Type 2 Diabetes?

Our cells and muscles use glucose to perform their functions. Exercise increases our energy usage, improving blood glucose control in diabetes patients (Colberg et al., 2016). Regular exercise can reduce our risk of developing type 2 diabetes and comorbidities. Medical professionals know that blood glucose management varies with each patient, which is why exercise recommendations should be tailored for the individual.

I've Been Diagnosed With Hypertension. Will Exercise Help?

Exercise can lower high blood pressure, but only if we maintain our fitness routine. Generally, 30 minutes of moderately intense physical activity per day is enough to make a positive impact on blood pressure (*10 drug-free ways to control high blood pressure*, n.d.). Regular exercise can potentially keep elevated blood pressure from turning into a more severe condition.

Is Exercise Safe for Cancer Survivors?

For most people, exercise before, during, and after cancer treatment is safe (*Physical Activity and the Person with Cancer*, 2022). Exercise can help us better cope with treatment side effects and may decrease our risk of developing new cancers. Make sure to consult your healthcare professional to ensure that your exercise plan matches your physical abilities and health status.

SAFETY TIPS

While the benefits may outweigh the risks, many people worry about their safety while exercising. Fortunately, there are ways to prevent troublesome situations from arising, giving you the safest possible experience. These guidelines should help:

- **Team Up:** When learning a new exercise, choose a partner to help you. They'll help you perfect your form, catch you if you lose your balance, and help you remain steady during the exercise.

- **Choose the Right Activity:** We should steer clear of activities that will worsen pre-existing conditions or that are a bad fit for our lifestyle and fitness goals. Your healthcare professional can point you in the right direction.

- **Start Slow:** Whether you are warming up for a workout session, or looking to increase the intensity of your fitness program, start slow! If we leap into strenuous activity too fast, we increase our likelihood of injury significantly. We need to have patience with our bodies and give them time to adjust to new activities. Introduce new exercises slowly, focusing on mastering form before increasing the intensity of the activity.

- *Gear Matters:* A safe environment and appropriate gear can go a long way in creating safe workout experiences. Try to maintain awareness of your surroundings and keep a bottle of water close at hand to rehydrate.

- *Seek Advice:* If you are suffering from chronic conditions (like chronic pain) ask your healthcare professional which physical activities are recommended for you.

- *Stop if You Feel Pain:* If an individual experiences pain or lightheadedness at any point during physical activity, it is advised to stop immediately. A healthcare professional should be consulted if the pain/lightheadedness persists.

This chapter hopefully addressed some general concerns you had about exercising. Many people know that they should be exercising more, but find the follow-through to be an obstacle. Overcoming this obstacle is precisely what we'll do in the next chapter.

CHAPTER 2

MINDSET MATTERS

False information in the fitness space often spreads through social media. A recent example of this includes a dance craze on TikTok. This unconventional dance claimed to be an ab workout and quickly became popular among youngsters, despite many experts' warnings that it is ineffective and dangerous. There's no doubt that misleading information can color the way we see fitness in our golden years, so let's help wipe the mindset slate clean by addressing some persistent myths.

- *"Exercising at my age? It's Pointless."* This could not be further from the truth. Our bodies are on a constant journey of change. Regular exercise keeps our muscles strong and flexible, making the body more resilient against frailty and other changes in our golden years. A regular fitness habit allows us to maintain and improve our mobility and quality of life. The beautiful thing about the human body is its ability to adapt. That means it is never pointless or too late to start a journey that will benefit us positively.

- *"If I exercise, I'll fall more!"* This concern is rooted in logic. The more we move, especially with balance issues, the higher the risk of falling and sustaining an injury. So, if we follow this train of thought, we'll end up moving less and leading a sedentary lifestyle. With our muscles weakened from the lack of movement, our risk of falling and sustaining injury increases. Our muscle mass tends to decline at a rate of three to eight percent per decade after our 30s (Volpi et al., 2004). Muscle decline is even higher in our 60s and contributes to disability in older adults. We need regular exercise to keep our muscles healthy, which will enable us to maintain our independence longer.

- *"I can't exercise with disabilities or health problems."* Disabilities and health concerns certainly place some parameters on the type of exercise we'll be able to do, but they do not necessarily preclude us from the activity. Seek guidance from a professional and respect your body's limitations. It is better to build on small gains, creating a healthy exercise habit that will encourage long-term benefits.

- *"I feel too weak or sore."* It is best to ease into activity when we feel weak or sore. Unless recommended by your doctor, it is generally safe to remain active. A balanced fitness plan helps us to manage pain and strengthens our bodies. Many people in their golden years can stem their decline in strength through regular physical activity (*Physical activity for seniors,* 2012).

GETTING INTO THE RIGHT HEADSPACE

Now that we've debunked some misleading myths, it is time to take a closer look at mindset. Some people associate exercise with the idea of sweating on the elliptical, while others think it is a solitary activity. Chances are, we've all had a New Year's resolution that went something like "exercise more and stay fit." The truth is, exercise is what you make of it. It can be a fun, engaging, and social activity. Those who make fitness a habit tend to personalize their workout routine by:

- Listening to music or an audiobook during the workout.
- Staying active throughout the day.
- Playing pickleball or doing tai chi.
- Watching television while on the treadmill or exercise bike.
- Walking instead of driving to nearby destinations, if safe or possible.

Physical activity can take many shapes! Activities that we enjoy keep us motivated and can help us commit to a balanced workout schedule much easier. Now that we are motivated to engage in an activity, we need to apply discipline. That means being committed and consistent to achieve the results you want. As you think about the results you'd like to achieve, consider the following:

- ***The Reason:*** The reasons we do something can be powerful sources of motivation, especially when we feel impatient with our fitness journey. Take a moment to consider why you started this journey. Maybe you wanted to feel more energetic. Or perhaps you wanted to manage your pain. There is no right or wrong answer here, our reasons are unique and personal.

- ***Planning:*** Write down your reason and plan ways for how you'll incorporate physical activity into your day. Planning takes the guesswork out and helps us mentally prepare for the task ahead. Having a written reminder can be a handy source of motivation as well.

- ***Accountability:*** Teaming up with a fitness buddy can go a long way in keeping us accountable and motivated.

- ***Rewarding Yourself:*** Whether you are celebrating a successful workout or achieving one of your fitness goals, rewarding yourself can be a great way to maintain motivation. Rewarding ourselves serves as a reminder that we are on a journey to develop a healthy relationship with our bodies. This includes developing a healthy relationship with food. This means that rewarding ourselves with that much-loved chocolate bar (or the tiny version thereof) may not always fall into our fitness plans. Exploring healthy, non-food reward alternatives will go a long way toward helping us change our body composition.

- ***Keeping Logs:*** Logging your workout can be a source of motivation in itself. Logging gives us a record of our progress, showing us exactly how much we've improved in a short period. Fitness apps for mobile devices often include exercise logs where we can track several items related to our workout including weight, workout duration, exercises performed, and the number of repetitions completed.

Nurturing Fitness as a Habit

A clear understanding of our reasons and how we'll go about becoming more active is key to making fitness a habit. The trick is to get into that headspace that encourages us to exercise voluntarily. Adopting a new habit is always tricky, but there are a few steps you can take that will help smooth things along.

- *"Go hard or go home" Is Terrible Advice. Ditch it.*

While it is a great attitude to have in endurance or high-adrenaline sports, it is not an approach we should adopt in our fitness routines. The athletes participating in these sports adopt this mentality to commit to big endeavors, like the Tour de France. But if we approach our daily workouts with this do-or-die mentality, we'll quickly become disenchanted and stop working out altogether. Ditching this mindset is a step in the right direction. Focus on small gains and listen to your body instead. The difference may surprise you!

- *Make it Fun!*

There are millions of people who find it difficult to stay motivated to exercise. That's because they are making a crucial mistake. Exercise is supposed to be fun, not torture. So, spend your time doing things that you enjoy. Whether it be tai chi, yoga, or regular golf outings, if you look forward to the activity, you'll be able to work out regularly.

- *Keep Goals Realistic*

Before starting a new fitness routine, it is a good idea to set a goal for yourself. Keep yourself from becoming overwhelmed by sticking to one small goal, along with a list of objectives (Blaszczak, 2016). That way, you'll be able to set realistic, achievable expectations for yourself.

- *Use Schedules*

Tying in with the idea of writing down our goals and logging out exercise, scheduling activities into our day can make accomplishing goals easier. Simply set a reminder on your mobile and don't cheat. The scheduling approach can prove particularly beneficial for chronic pain patients. Research shows that multiple short exercise sessions give us the same benefits as one long workout session would (*Exercise for Chronic Pain Management - 7 Tips*, 2022). Try adding 10 minutes of morning stretches followed by light cardio. Repeat the process again at lunchtime, and wind down at bedtime with light stretches. Breaking up a 30-minute routine like this can be an effective way to stay active.

- ***Experiment and Make It Social***

Deciding on a fitness routine does not have to tie you to a gym. There are times when being at the gym can be a hindrance to our physical fitness. When this happens, fill the time with an enjoyable physical activity instead. There are many different kinds of activities that keep us moving without feeling like a workout, for example, dancing and walking tours. Bring a friend along and make it a social affair. It is a great way to remain accountable and committed to your plans.

- ***Get the Chores Done***

Whether it is walking the dog or sweeping the deck, they count as physical activities. It is best to prepare for strenuous activities with a warm-up and maintain awareness of your posture and joint alignment during the activity. Take note of any sore muscles the day after. This will help us better prepare our muscles the next time we engage in that activity.

- ***Practice Mindfulness***

Mindfulness involves paying attention to our breathing, how our body moves, and how we feel during activities. The goal is to heighten our self-awareness in an attempt to prevent injury.

Now that we're armed with tips on how to make fitness a habit, it's time to set those goals. Goals are divided into short and long-term categories. Short-term goals refer to tasks we'll be able to accomplish in a week or two. Maybe you want to improve your energy levels or bike a couple of miles. After you've decided on the goal, pick your reward. Select something that will keep you motivated to achieve the goal. Short-term goals can be used to nurture the approach we would like to take in our fitness journey, and are vital in staying motivated.

Long-term goals generally build on our short-term goals. If, for example, your long-term goal is to go for a 10-mile hike, structure your short-term goals to support this. Remember to keep your goals realistic, and you'll be surprised by the outcomes. Now that we're better mentally prepared for the rigors of a fitness routine, it is time to dive into an important but very neglected aspect of fitness: The warm-up.

CHAPTER 3

NURTURING FLEXIBILITY–WARMING UP AND COOLING DOWN

Warming up and cooling down are the foundations on which a successful fitness journey is built. Yet, these brief periods at the start and end of our routines are often neglected or hurried through. Many people skip the warm-up to get to the heart of their workout, but this is a bad practice. When we fail to properly prepare the body for a strenuous activity, we are flirting with injury. Not only does the risk of serious injury increase, but the results from our fitness program will not be optimal. Skipping the warm-up only results in wasting our time and energy. Warming up allows our heart rate to gradually increase, supplying our muscles with enough oxygen in the process (*Why Warming Up and Cooling Down is Important*, 2016). It is a necessary step to warm and prepare the body for coming activity and can prevent many injuries.

As a rule of thumb, start every workout session with a warm-up. The warm-up should last 5–10 minutes and include stretches and mild activity (like walking in place). End every session with 5–10 minutes of stretching. This allows our heart rate to slowly return to normal, reducing the likelihood of dizzy spells afterward.

Flexibility comes into play because it increases our joint mobility and range of motion. As we journey through life, our muscle strength and flexibility decline. This is one of the biggest reasons why getting up from a chair becomes more challenging in our golden years. A decline in flexibility affects our balance and posture and can place us at risk of experiencing chronic pain (Bilodeau, 2019). Strengthening regularly keeps our muscles flexible and strong, enabling them to better support our joints. This helps to eliminate many sources of mild pains and aches. Not all stretches are the same, but we'll explore the difference between static and dynamic stretches below.

- *Static Stretches:* These are stretches that place tension on a certain muscle group. Static stretches are typically held for 10–30 seconds. Many hamstring stretches fall into this category. These stretches are best used in the cooldown.

- *Dynamic Stretches:* These typically form part of our warm-up routine and use a range of motions to engage many muscle groups. These stretches are typically gentler versions of the main workout and are performed at a slower palace. Yoga is a well-known example of dynamic stretching.

Static and dynamic stretches can help us get the most out of our workout session, but there are still a few things we need to keep in mind. Two sins, if you will.

- *Sin One: Holding Our Breath*

This happens more often than you think! When we are focused on mastering form, it can be easy to hold our breath during a workout. Doing so is a bad idea. Holding our breath in this situation places the body under stress, making our muscles tight. We want to maintain a steady breathing pattern throughout our workout session, so our muscles are relaxed, oxygenated, and performing well. The simplest way to do this is to time our movements with our breath. We inhale with certain movements and exhale with others.

- *Sin Two: Going Through the Motions*

When we are stretching, it is best to avoid jerky movements. We want to move slowly and steadily, remaining in full control of our movements. When we rush through the warm-up, we risk muscle spasms and discomfort.

When stretching, it is advised to only go as far as you comfortably can. If you feel pain, stop immediately. If you feel at any point in your workout that something is not right, err on the side of caution and stop. Never push yourself beyond your limits; it is only an invitation for pain. "Pain" does not include the slow, gentle burn we may experience when holding a stretch for 10–30 seconds. As our bodies adapt to our fitness routines, we can start to customize our workouts. We can increase the duration of some poses, but for now, it is best to aim for 30 seconds.

Structuring Your Warm-up and Cooldown

Warming up and cooling down follow a general structure. For a warm-up, it is best to do 5–10 minutes of mildly intense activity (walking or light cardio). The idea is to gently elevate our heart rates, warming our bodies, without overusing our muscles. Follow up with a few stretches, targeting the areas of your body that you intend to exercise. Or simply do a general stretch of your whole body.

Cooldowns are structured similarly. Generally, we'll spend 5–10 minutes on cardio, after which stretching follows. These stretches typically target the muscles we've just worked out, helping to reduce pain and stiffness in the days that follow.

STRETCHES FOR YOUR UPPER-BODY

In this section, we'll delve into the various stretches you can include in your routine. These stretches will target the upper body. Don't worry, I'll guide you with instructions on how to perform each stretch safely.

Neck

Painful neck? The good news is that stretching can help to provide temporary pain relief (Ylinen et al., 2007). When stretching your neck, resist the urge to push through the pain. Pain is usually a sign that something is wrong. Our alignment could be off, or something else might be at play. Listen to your body, and never ignore the cues it gives.

Neck Extension Stretch

- Sit tall in your chair. Draw your shoulders down and away from the ears.

- Gently tip your head backward, as far as you comfortably can. This should be a controlled movement. Hold the stretch for 10 seconds and gently bring your head back. Repeat for as many sets and reps as needed.

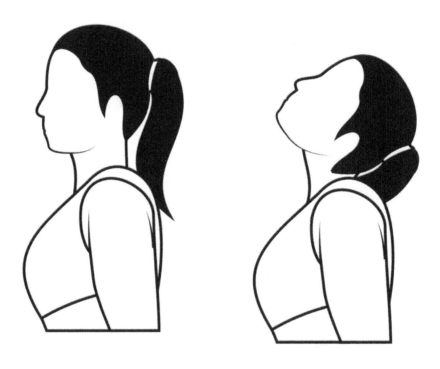

Figure 1: Neck Extension Stretch

Neck Flexion Stretch

- Sit upright in your chair. Draw your shoulders away from your ears.

- Slowly drop your chin towards your chest, stretching the back of your neck. You can increase the intensity of the stretch by applying gentle pressure with your hands. Place them at the back of our heads to deepen the stretch. Only deepen the stretch if you feel comfortable doing it.

- Hold the stretch for 10 seconds and gently bring your head upright. Repeat as many times as needed.

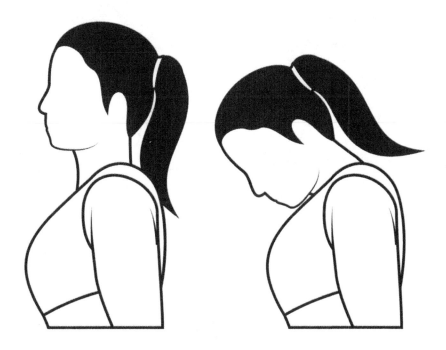

Figure 2: Neck Flexion Stretch

Neck Rotation Stretch

- Sit tall in a chair. As per usual, draw your shoulders away from your ears.

- Turn your head to look over your shoulder as far as you comfortably can. Hold the position for 10 seconds.

- Return your head to the starting position and repeat on the opposite side. Complete as many sets and reps as desired.

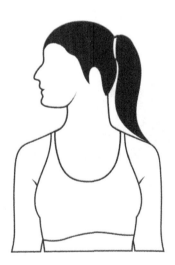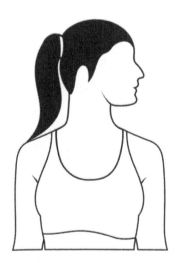

Figure 3: Neck Rotation Stretch

Levator Scapula Stretch

- Sitting with hunched shoulders usually causes pain in this muscle group. This stretch can help to ease the soreness.

- Sit up straight in your chair. Draw your shoulders away from your ears.

- Stabilize the shoulder blade of the side you are stretching with your hand. Place it behind the shoulder.

- Turn your head 45 degrees to one side and lower your chin. Try looking at your knee, you should feel a stretch. If you want to increase the intensity of the stretch, you'll need to rest your hand on the back of your head. From there, apply gentle pressure to increase the intensity of the stretch.

- Hold the stretch for 10 seconds and repeat on the opposite side.

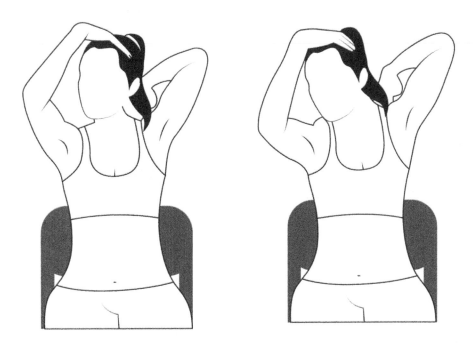

Figure 4: Levator Scapula Stretch

Neck Side Stretch

- Sit tall and straight in your chair. Draw your shoulders back and down, taking them away from the ears.

- Gently bend your neck, bringing an ear closer to your shoulder. Try to keep your shoulders tell. If you want to deepen the stretch, apply gentle pressure to the side of your head with your hand.

- Hold the stretch for 10 seconds. Gently release the stretch and repeat on the opposite side. Complete as many sets and reps as desired.

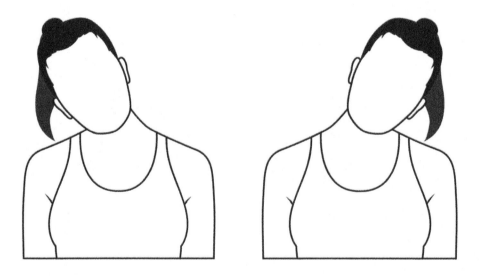

Figure 5: Neck Side Stretch

Chin Drop

- This exercise can be done in a seated or standing position. Bring your arms in front of you, elbows and palms facing each other. Gently turn your hands, facing your palms towards you. From here, place your palms on your head.

- Without applying any pressure with your hands, slowly lower your chin and bring it closer to your chest. Hold the position for 10–30 seconds.

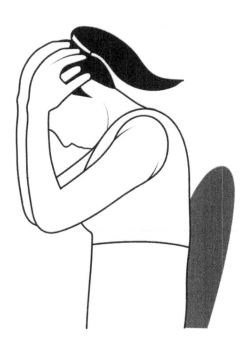

Figure 6: Chin Drop

Arms and Shoulders

Keeping your arms and shoulders mobile is a key factor in ensuring your independence. Just think of activities like getting dressed or reaching for items off a shelf.

Arm Opener

- Stand tall with your feet shoulder-width apart. Keep your toes and knees pointing forward.

- Move your hands behind your back and interlace your fingers. Let your fingers rest against your tailbone, keeping the knuckles facing outward.

- Keep your body straight as you slowly raise your arms away from the tailbone. Keep your fingers interlaced as you raise your arms as high as is comfortable. Hold the position for 10–30 seconds, before gently returning your hands to their starting position.

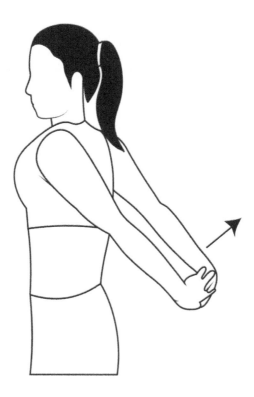

Figure 7: Arm Opener

Shoulder and Arm Stretch

- Hold a towel or strap in one hand and drape it behind your back.

- Reach for the other end of the strap with your other hand, gently pulling on it behind your back until you feel a stretch. Hold the stretch for 10–30 seconds and repeat on the opposite side.

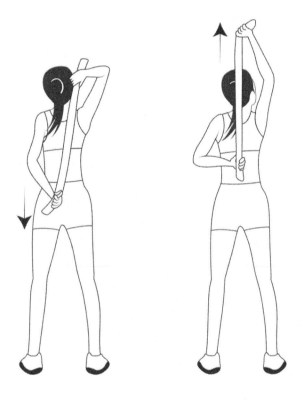

Figure 8: Shoulder and Arm Stretch

Overhead Stretch

- Sit upright in your chair. Keep your back straight and core lightly engaged. Next, interlace your fingers and gently raise your arms to bring them overhead. The idea is to keep the arms straight with the palms facing the ceiling.

- Hold the pose for 10–30 seconds, before gently lowering your arms to release the stretch.

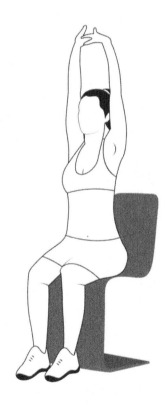

Figure 9: Overhead Stretch

Shoulder Cross-Arm Stretch

- Sit tall and draw your shoulders away from the ears.

- Straighten one arm out in front of your chest. Use your other arm to gently hug the arm across your body, increasing the intensity of the stretch. Hold the position for 10–30 seconds and repeat on the opposite side.

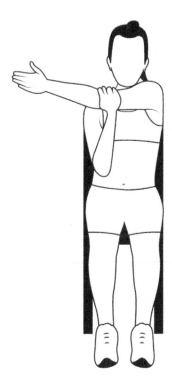

Figure 10: Shoulder Cross-Arm Stretch

Chest

Chest stretches target the upper front part of our torsos, where the pectoralis muscles are housed. These muscles play a central role in good posture, shoulder mobility, neck movement, and the pushing or pulling of heavy objects. Tight chest muscles often lead to pain in the neck and shoulder and can hamper our ability to lift things. It is advised to perform chest stretches as part of your warm-up or cooldown routine to improve posture and overall upper-body mobility.

Standing Chest Stretch

- Stand tall, with your feet hip distance apart and your toes facing forward. Keep your core lightly engaged.

- Next, extend both arms side wards with your palms facing forward. Gently reach back with your hands. You should feel a stretch develop across your chest and arms. Hold the position for 10–30 seconds.

- Consider propping your hands against a wall if you have a hard time holding your arms up. Simply place your hand on a wall and step forward until you feel a stretch. Hold the stretch for 10–30 seconds and repeat on the other side. Be careful not to overdo things with this stretch.

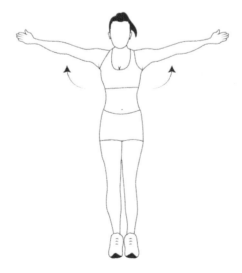

Figure 11: Standing Chest Stretch

Seated Chest Stretch

- Sit straight in your chair and draw your shoulders away from the ears.

- Extend your arms straight in front of you, keeping them parallel to the floor. If you have a hard time keeping them parallel, lower them to a 45-degree angle instead. Next, bring your arms to the side, going as far back as you can. Squeeze the shoulder blades while maintaining your upright posture.

- Hold the posture for 10–30 seconds.

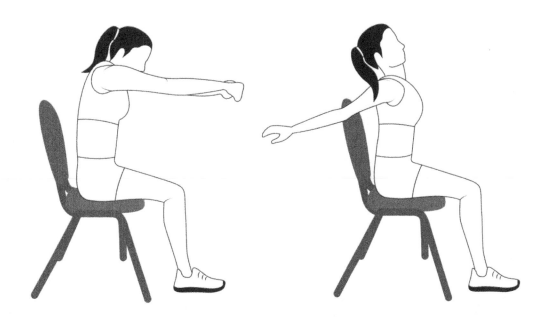

Figure 12: Seated Chest Stretch

Back

Regular stretching of the back can help to reduce tension in the muscles that support the spine, alleviating pain and improving our range of motion (Gopez, 2017). It should be noted that if we experience pain that lasts longer than three months, it can take several weeks for a fitness regimen to successfully reduce pain.

Thoracic Extension

- As per usual, sit tall in your chair and draw your shoulders away from the ears. Rest your hands behind your head, ideally with the fingertips touching. Be mindful to keep your posture erect and your core engaged.

- From here, slowly extend your upper back over the chair. Hold the stretch for 10–30 seconds and gently bring your body upright again.

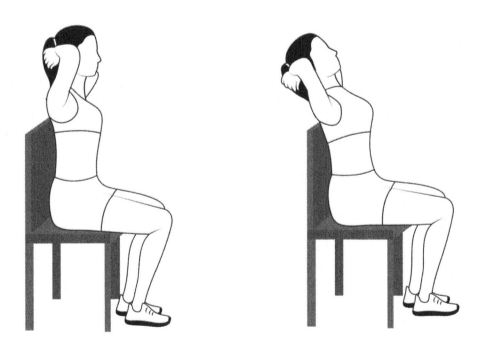

Figure 13: Thoracic Extension

Thoracic Rotation

- Draw your shoulders back from the ears and sit upright in your chair. Be sure to rest your weight on the triangle of your tailbone and sitz bones whenever sitting up straight. Now we'll add rotation. With arms crossed over the chest, rotate until you feel the stretch. You'll need to lead with your arms to achieve this.

- Hold the stretch for 10–30 seconds and repeat on the other side.

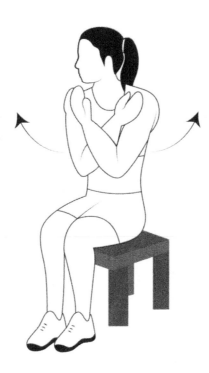

Figure 14: Thoracic Rotation

Rhomboids Stretch

- Assume an upright seated posture, with shoulders away from the ears. Interlace your fingers. Now, push your palms outwards and away from yourself.

- Next, you'll need to raise your arms, keeping them parallel to the floor. Push your hands out as far as you can. The trick is to keep your posture straight, that way you'll feel your shoulder blades stretch.

- Hold the stretch for 10–30 seconds and gently reverse your movements to release the stretch.

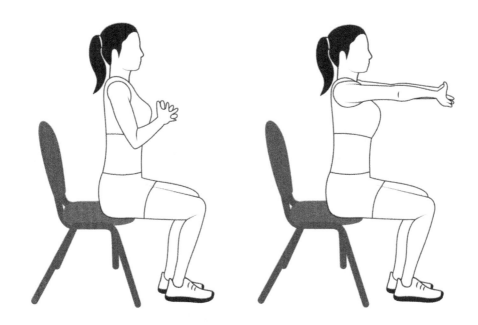

Figure 15: Rhomboids Stretch

Wrist

When was the last time you stretched your wrists? Our wrists are in use throughout the day. Whether we are writing, typing, scrolling, lifting a grocery bag, or cooking dinner, our wrists remain busy! Stiff, inflexible wrists can make a lot of our daily tasks more challenging to complete, but a few simple stretches can help to turn things around.

Wrist Extension Stretch

- Draw your shoulders away from your ears and straighten your spine.

- Reach one arm in front of your body. The palm should be facing down, fingers pointed up.

- Using the other hand, gently apply pressure to bend the wrist. Your arm should remain straight the entire time. Hold the stretch for 10–30 seconds and repeat on the opposite side.

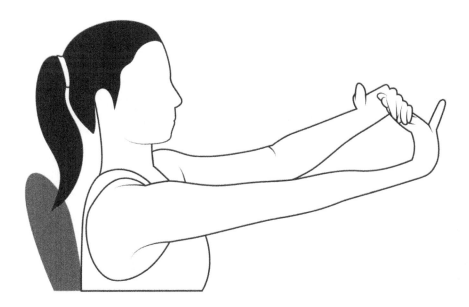

Figure 16: Wrist Extension Stretch

Wrist Flexion Stretch

- Sitting tall in your chair, reach with one arm straight in front of you. Your palm should be facing down, and your fingers pointed upwards. Now relax your wrist, allowing it to soften.

- Using the other hand, apply gentle pressure to the back of the hand, bending the wrist downward. Keep your arm straight while doing so. Maintain the stretch for 10–30 seconds and repeat on the opposite side.

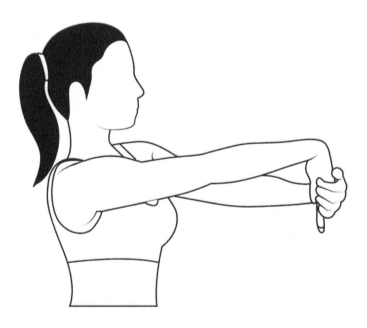

Figure 17: Wrist Flexion Stretch

STRETCHES FOR YOUR LOWER-BODY

Standing Stretches for Legs

Tight quads, hamstrings, and hip flexors are common causes of low back pain (*Importance of Stretching,* n.d.). That's because short, tight muscles alter the way we move, which can contribute to low back pain. Regular stretching can make a difference in many cases.

Downward Dog

- You'll need to get onto all fours for this one. Position your hands shoulder-width apart. Your knees and feet should be kept hip-width apart.

- Slowly raise your knees, straightening your legs as much as possible. Keep your heels planted on the floor. Your back should be straight, ideally forming an inverted V-shape with your legs.

- Relax your neck and spine as you maintain the pose for 10–30 seconds. Slowly reverse your movements to disengage from the stretch.

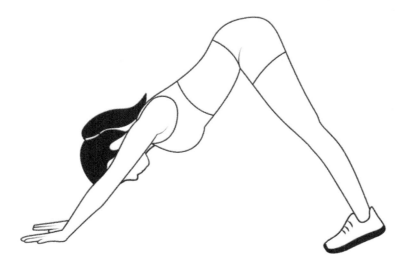

Figure 18: Downward Dog

Standing Hamstring Stretch

- Stand tall next to a chair. Use the chair to steady yourself if you need to.

- Step one foot forward. Be mindful to keep your knees straight and heels touching the floor the whole time. Keep your knees soft and square your hips.

- Gently lean forward, hinging at the hips. You should feel a stretch in the back of your leg. Hold the stretch for 10–30 seconds and repeat on the opposite side.

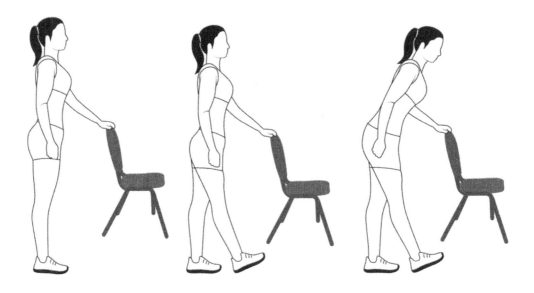

Figure 19: Standing Hamstring Stretch

Calf Stretch

- Grip the backrest of a sturdy chair and stand tall. Take a minute to position your toes, making sure that they point forward at all times.

- Carefully place one foot behind you.

- Bend your leading knee towards the chair. Your heels should remain on the ground.

- Hold the stretch for 10–30 seconds and repeat on the other side.

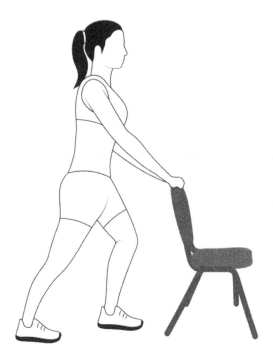

Figure 20: Calf Stretch

Hip Abductor Stretch

- Stand tall. From here, choose your left or right foot and step out to the side. Keep your toes pointing outwards.

- Shift your weight to one foot, bending at the knee. This will stretch the inner thigh of your straight leg. Use a chair to steady yourself if needed.

- Hold the stretch for 10–30 seconds and repeat with the other leg.

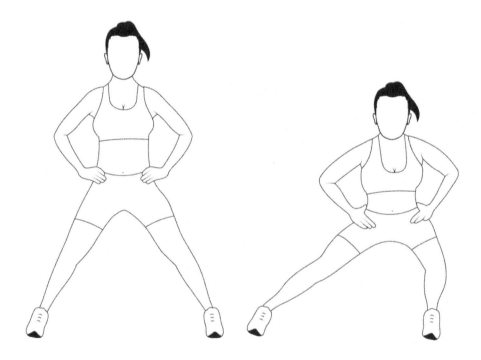

Figure 21: Hip Abductor Stretch

Standing Quadricep Stretch

- Stand next to a sturdy chair. Use one hand to steady yourself during the stretch.

- Keep your back straight as you bring one foot behind you. Reach down and hold on to it with your free hand. Your posture must remain straight. Bring your knees next to each other and hold the stretch.

- After 10–30 seconds, release your foot gently and repeat on the opposite side.

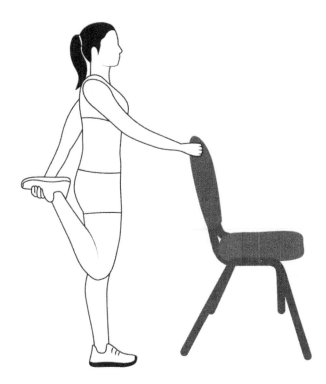

Figure 22: Standing Quadricep Stretch

Seated Stretches for Legs

Regular stretching can help steady our gait! Research found that a regular stretching program can be effective at addressing some variables influencing our gait (Cristopoliski et al., 2009). This makes regular stretching a very effective way to reverse some of the age-related changes we may experience along the way. So take a few minutes and try these seated stretches. Your body will thank you later.

Hip Flexion Stretch

- Sit tall in your chair, with your shoulders drawn away from the ears.

- Slowly raise one leg, bringing it to your chest. Bend your knee and hug the leg gently. Hold the stretch for 10–30 seconds and repeat on the opposite side.

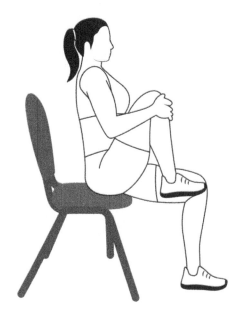

Figure 23: Hip Flexion Stretch

Hip Lateral Rotation Stretch

- Sit tall, towards the front of your chair. Hold on to the seat of your chair firmly.

- Extend your legs, slowly crossing one over the other. Slide the heel up the shin and over the knee. This should be a slow and controlled movement.

- Keep your back straight as you bend the opposite leg now. Rest your hands on your shins and maintain the pose for 10–30 seconds. If you want to deepen the stretch, simply lean forward. Gently reverse your movements to release the stretch and repeat on the opposite side.

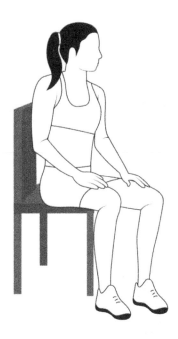

Figure 24: Hip Lateral Rotation Stretch - Part 1

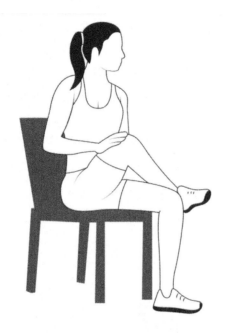

Figure 25: Hip Lateral Rotation Stretch - Part 2

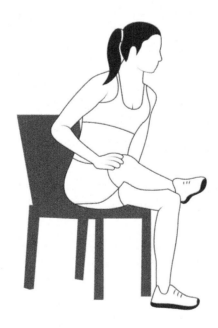

Figure 26: Hip Lateral Rotation Stretch - Part 3

Seated Hamstring Stretch

- Sit towards the front of your chair. Slowly extend one leg. Rest your hands on the bent leg.

- As you extend your leg, keep it straight and point your toes upward. Keep your back straight. Hold the position for 10–30 seconds and change legs.

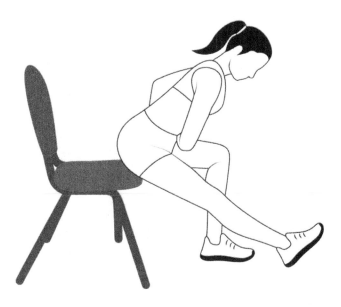

Figure 27: Seated Hamstring Stretch

Abductor Stretch

- Sit tall, towards the front of a sturdy chair.

- Move one leg out to the side. Ensure that your toes are firmly grounded and facing forward. You should feel a stretch in the inner thigh of the straight leg.

- To increase the intensity of the stretch, simply bend forward. Hold the stretch for 10–30 seconds and switch legs. Make sure to keep your back straight throughout the exercise.

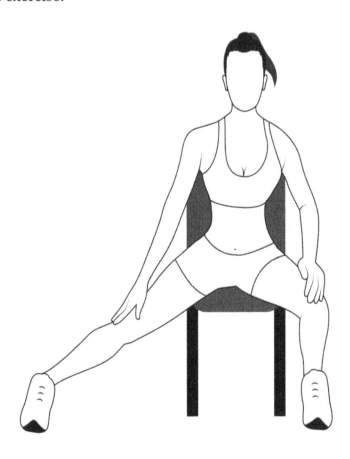

Figure 28: Abductor Stretch

Ankle Stretch

- Sit tall in your chair. Slowly move your feet up and down. Hold each position for 10–30 seconds.

- Now slowly mow your feet side to side, once again holding the stretches for 10–30 seconds.

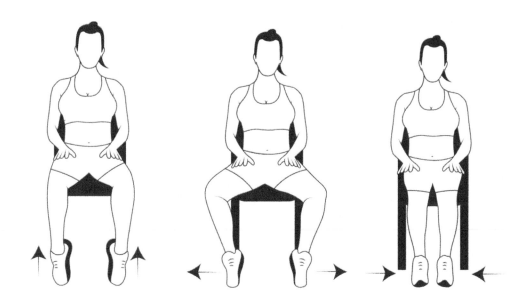

Figure 29: Ankle Stretch

Lying Stretches for Legs

Don't feel like standing or sitting? We've got you covered! The stretches in this section are done while lying down and provide the same benefits as the stretches mentioned in previous sections. Having a variety of stretches at our disposal helps us work out muscles from different angles, giving us better results. If you don't feel comfortable lying down on the floor, feel free to perform these stretches lying on your bed.

Lying Hamstring Stretch

- Lie comfortably on your back. Keep your shoulders and hips firmly on the floor.

- Extend one leg. It should be perpendicular to your body. Next, you'll need to reach for and grab the back of your thigh.

- Be mindful that your hips and other legs remain on the floor. Gently pull your leg towards your chest and maintain the stretch for 10–30 seconds. Release and switch sides.

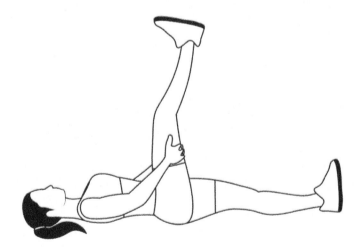

Figure 30: Lying Hamstring Stretch

Lying Quadricep Stretch

- Lie on your side. Bring your foot behind you and reach for it.

- Take hold of your foot. Keep your back straight and gently pull until you feel a stretch. Maintain the stretch for 10–30 seconds before gently releasing. Repeat on the opposite side.

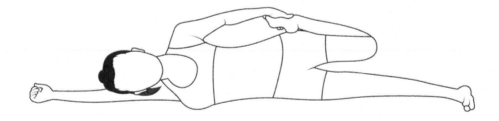

Figure 31: Lying Quadricep Stretch

Lying Hip Stretch

- Lie comfortably on your back with your shoulders and hips firmly on the floor. Move one knee out to the side, and rest your foot against your other leg.

- Now gently push down with the bent knee, and you should feel a stretch. Hold the stretch for 10–30 seconds and repeat on the opposite side.

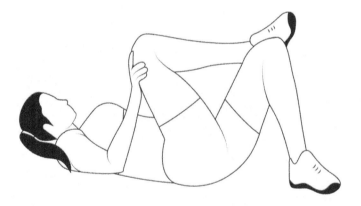

Figure 32: Lying Hip Stretch

Seated Stretches for the Lower Back

Back pain is the second most common reason we visit the doctor, according to the American Chiropractic Association (Stelter, 2014). This means that keeping our postural muscles in good form can help us save on doctors' bills in the long run. The stretches in this section will help to keep the lower back flexible and strong.

Lumbar Flexion

- Sit upright in your chair with your shoulders drawn away from the ears. Firmly plant your feet in front of you and rest your hands on your knees.

- Slowly slide your hands down the outsides of your legs to your feet. Hinge at the hips as you bend forward.

- Hold the stretch for 10–30 seconds and gently reverse your movements to release the stretch.

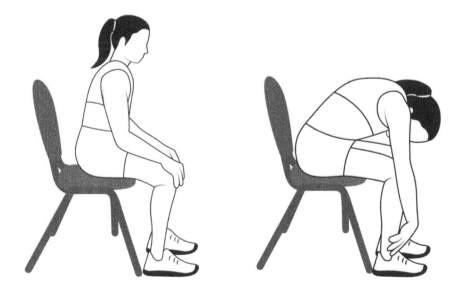

Figure 33: Lumbar Flexion Stretch

Lumbar Side Stretch

- Assume an upright seated position with your shoulders away from the ears.

- Keeping your posture erect, gently bend at the waist to the right. Reach overhead with your left arm.

- Hold the stretch for 10–30 seconds. Gently reverse your movements to come out of the stretch and repeat on the left.

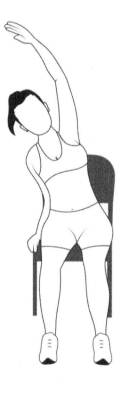

Figure 34: Lumbar Side Stretch

Lumbar Extension

- Sit tall in the middle of a sturdy chair. Rest your hands on the small of your back.

- Gently lean back, applying gentle pressure to your hands for a lower back stretch.

- Hold the stretch for 10–30 seconds.

All warmed up? Fantastic! Now we get to the fun part of this guide: The practical side. The chapters ahead contain many exercises that hold the power to transform our health!

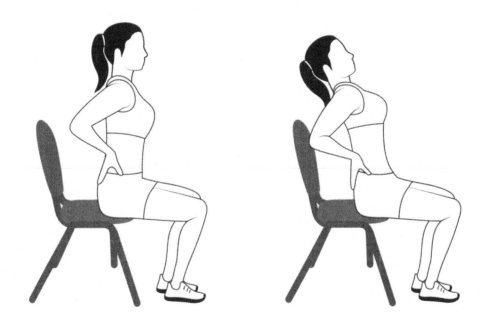

Figure 35: Lumbar Extension

CHAPTER 4

MASTERING CORE EXERCISES

You've probably heard talk about why our core muscles are important. From making everyday movement possible to enabling us to hold Pilates and Yoga poses, the core plays a crucial role in our daily lives. A strong core stabilizes and balances us and helps to improve our posture, reducing the risk of injury and pain (Carter, 2022). A strong core can make a difference in your golf game, but when it comes to exercising, many people fall into the "situps only" trap. They erroneously believe that strong abs will result in a strong core, but this is only half the picture. That is why we'll focus exclusively on the core and the exercises that will strengthen these muscles in this chapter.

MORE THAN A SIX PACK

Let's start by gaining a deeper understanding of the core. It is the group of trunk and hip muscles that surround the hip, spine, and abdominal viscera (*Core Muscles*, n.d.). In less accurate terms, the "core" can be described as everything located above your legs and between your arms (except for the neck and head). That means the core makes up a considerably large part of our bodies! The core is essential for proper load distribution along the spine and pelvis, this is why weak core muscles and a painful lower back often share a direct relationship.

Multiple muscle groups create the core, including the traverse abdominis, obliques, pelvic floor muscles, diaphragm, rectus abdominis, and abs. Let's not forget the smaller core muscles including the lats, traps, and (to the surprise of many) our glutes (Thieme, 2021). Each of these muscles plays a role in our daily functioning and movement, working cohesively to stabilize and power our bodies and limbs. Essentially this means that the stronger your core is, the better you'll be able to avoid potential injury and pain. That being said, let's take a closer look at some key muscle groups in our core.

- **Gluteus Maximus and Medius:** This muscle goes by many names. Some call it the *"gluteus maximus"* while others refer to this meaty muscle less scientifically as the *'tush'*. Whatever your naming preference, this muscle group helps us to stand up straight, walk and climb stairs. If the buttocks are the powerhouse behind these movements, then the gluteus medius is the stabilizer. This group of muscles are located on the side of our buttocks and helps to keep our knees steady while walking, standing, or climbing stairs (Galloway, 2022).

- **Rectus Abdominis:** These are the muscles' fitness fiends and gym rats often exercise in their pursuit of a six-pack. This muscle is located between the ribs and our pubic bone, and its chief function is to help us flex and bend our bodies (*Abdominal muscles,* 2012).

- **External and Internal Obliques:** Our obliques (located on the sides of the torso) help the body to twist and bend. Sometimes a layer of fat develops on top of the obliques, which earned them the "love handle" nickname. It can be challenging to lose that unflattering layer of fat on top of the obliques, but doing so contributes to a stronger core and a well-trained look.

- **Transversus Abdominis:** The deepest abdominal muscle is responsible for helping us breathe and stabilizing the pelvis and lower back (Edwards & Ward, 2022).

Training your core consistently does so much more than help us walk with a steadier gait. A strong core is vital to improving our posture and reducing back pain. On top of this, a well-trained core can help to increase our mobility, balance, and coordination, lending strength to our workouts.

Upping the Ante

When starting a core workout (or any fitness program, for that matter), remember to take it easy! Start slow and concentrate on feeling your muscles contract. Gradually, as you gain strength and experience, increase the number of repetitions and sets to continue challenging your muscles.

Let's say you've decided to do five supermans twice a week as part of your fitness routine. Over time (anywhere from two to six weeks), you might notice that the exercise is not challenging you as much. In fact, you are hardly feeling it! That's because our bodies are quick to adapt. When this happens, it may become necessary to increase the reps or duration that an exercise is performed.

Core exercises might bring the classic sit-up and crunch to mind, but these exercises should be avoided. Most of the time, people perform these exercises wrong, training their hip flexors instead and placing unnecessary pressure on the neck.

CORE EXERCISES

Try to perform 5–10 repetitions of each exercise, building up to a daily practice. The entire core workout should take 10 minutes to complete, so you can easily slip in some core strengthening work during the day.

Seated Forward Roll-Ups

- Sit tall in a chair. Extend your legs, flexing your feet towards your body. Your heels should be resting on the floor.

- Reach your arms in front of your body. Be careful to keep your posture straight as you curl your chin towards the chest.

- Now for the tricky part: Exhale and roll your torso up and over, timing the movement to your breath. Your legs should remain straight and your core engaged.

- Slowly reach for your toes, going as far as you comfortably can. Once you've reached maximum extension, gently roll back to your starting position. Repeat the movement slowly and avoid rushing through the motion. The key is to remain mindful of your movements and use your abs to lift and lower yourself.

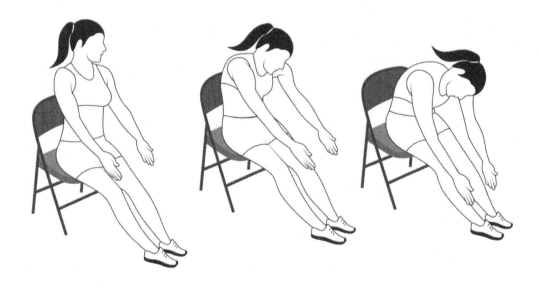

Figure 36: Seated Forward Roll-Ups

Seated Side Bends

- Sit tall in a sturdy chair. Plant your feet firmly on the floor with your toes pointed forward.

- Raise your right arm, bringing your hand to the side of your head. Maintain your upright posture and inhale deeply.

- On the exhale, bend gently at the waist, lowering your left arm towards the floor. Inhale as you return to the starting position. Complete as many reps as desired and repeat on the opposite side.

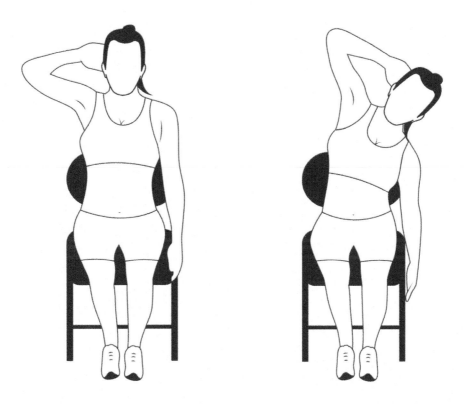

Figure 37: Seated Side Bends

Seated Leg Lifts

- Sit up straight in a sturdy chair. Straighten your right leg, but keep the left leg bent.

- Engage your core and gently raise the right leg as high as you can manage. The key here is to maintain straightness in your leg and back.

- Hold the pose briefly, before gently returning your right foot to the floor. Complete as many reps and sets as desired.

- Repeat the exercise on the left.

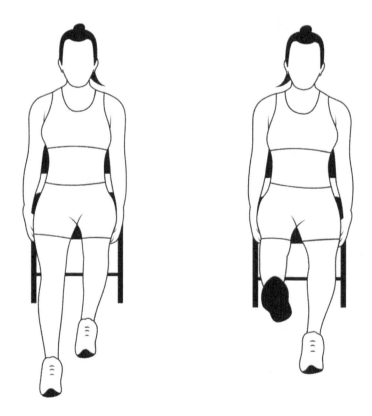

Figure 38: Seated Leg Lifts

Seated Leg Taps

- Sit tall in a chair with your feet firmly planted on the floor. Grip the sides of your seat to steady yourself.

- Engage your core as you steadily raise both legs and tap your feet on the floor.

- Rest your feet by pulling your legs under the chair and repeat the exercise as many times as desired.

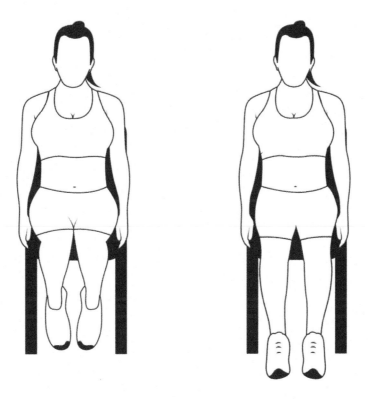

Figure 39: Seated Leg Taps

Forearm Planks

- You'll need to lie face-down for this one. Keep your forearms grounded and elbows under the shoulders. Engage your core and press through your forearms, palms, and toes to lift your body from the floor. Your body should form a straight line.

- Hold the pose for 10–30 seconds and gently lower yourself to the floor to release. If you feel pressure in your lower back, use your knees to provide support.

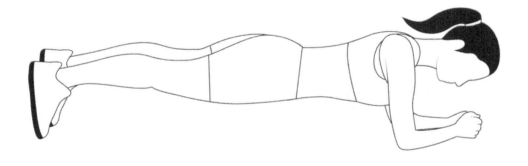

Figure 40: Forearm Planks

Superman

- Lie face-down, keeping your legs comfortably together. Reach overhead with your arms and tighten your abs and upper back, drawing your body into a gentle arch.

- Now lift your arms and legs off the ground simultaneously. Be careful not to stiffen your neck or shoulders. Hold the pose briefly before gently lowering yourself to the ground in a slow and controlled fashion.

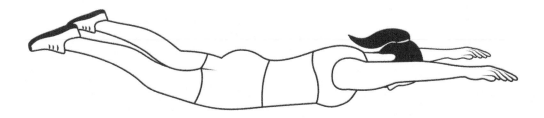

Figure 41: Superman

Glute Bridges

- Lie on your back with your knees bent and feet firmly planted on the floor. Your feet should be hip-distance apart.

- Now comes the tricky part: Engage your abs and use your glutes to lift your hips from the floor. Hold the pose for 10–30 seconds before returning your body to the floor slowly.

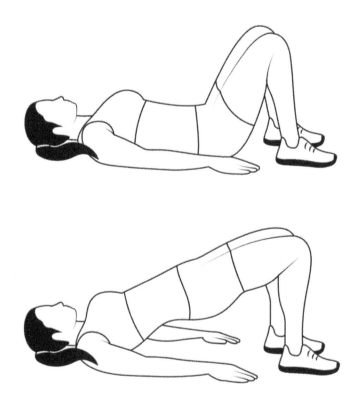

Figure 42: Glute Bridges

Wood Chops

- Stand tall with your feet hip-width apart. Move your arms in front of your body and hold your hands. Tighten your core as you raise your arms above your head towards the right.

- Exhale and slowly bring your arms across your body towards the left hip to 'chop'.

- On the inhale, raise your arms to the starting point. Repeat as many times as desired and switch sides.

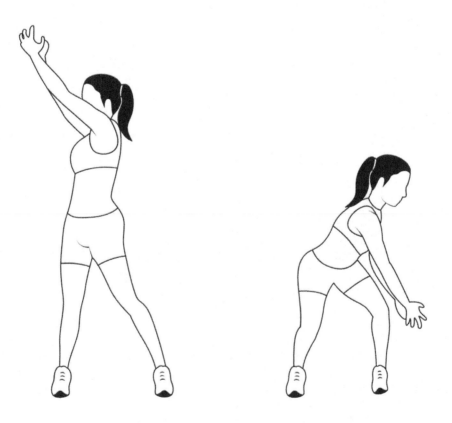

Figure 43: Wood Chops

Deadbug

- Lie on your back. Lift your feet from the floor and bend your knees to form a 90-degree angle. Reach with both arms towards the ceiling. This is the 'base' position.

- Now pull your belly in towards your spine and lower one foot to the floor. When your foot touches the floor, gently return it to the base position. Repeat as many times as desired and copy with the other leg.

- If the exercise is proving too hard, you can raise your arm above your head instead of lowering your legs. On the other hand, if you feel up for a challenge, try doing an arm and the opposing leg at the same time.

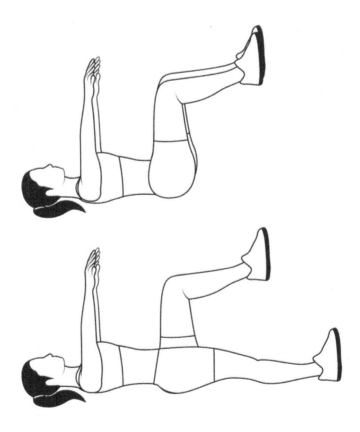

Figure 44: Deadbug – Basic

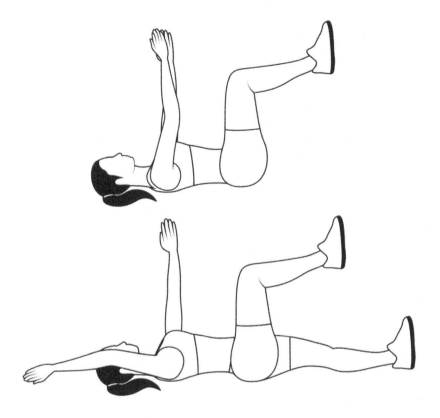

Figure 45: Deadbug - Advanced

Give these exercises a chance, and you might discover that your core is feeling a lot stronger and more stable, giving you a solid foundation to tackle the next portion of your fitness program.

CHAPTER 5

TRAINING THE UPPER BODY

A strong upper body can positively impact our physical activities by improving coordination, helping the body burn more calories, building endurance, and reducing artery damage that is linked to blood pressure, cholesterol, and blood sugar problems (*Benefits of Increasing Upper Body Strength*, 2021). Training the upper body shouldn't be confused with lifting weights, cross-training, or weighted pull-ups. While these forms of exercise target and strengthen the upper body, we can easily and safely exercise the upper body using nothing but our body weight and simple household items. The upper body is composed of several muscle groups, so let's take a closer look at them.

- *Deltoids:* The deltoids are located close to the surface of our skin, wrapping the shoulder joint. The base of the deltoid connects to the shoulder blade and collarbone, while the point of the muscle connects to the side of the humerus (*Deltoid Muscles: What Are They, Anatomy, Location & Function*, 2021). Exercising these muscles results in defined shoulders.

- *Pectoralis Major and Minor:* Our pectoralis major covers much of the font of the chest and helps us to push, rotate and move our arms across the body. The pectoralis minor is a stabilizing muscle and helps us to fine-tune movements between the ribs and shoulder blades.

- **Rotator Cuff:** The rotator cuff is separated into four muscles, each works in harmony with the other to lend our shoulders' stability when we move and lift objects. Keeping our rotator cuff flexible through exercising is crucial to maintain our full range of motion in the shoulder.

- **Biceps and Triceps:** The biceps is responsible for flexing the elbow. It is also the muscle we use to turn our palms upwards. Our triceps takes up the entire underside of our upper arm, and its main job is to extend the elbow. When one neglects their biceps and triceps, their arms become weak and shoulder mobility can be impacted.

- **Scapula:** Several muscle groups come together to stabilize the shoulder blade region, ensuring that the area remains flexible, mobile, and pain-free.

- **Forearms:** These muscles run from the wrist to the elbow. Don't let the relatively small size of the forearm fool you, there's plenty of muscle at work there! Their muscles play a role in the strength and flexibility of our hands, elbows, and wrists.

- **Latissimus Dorsi:** This is a broad, flat muscle that takes up much of the lower posterior thorax (Jeno & Varacallo, 2021). These muscles can pull up our body weight, and neglecting this area can lead to difficulty in raising our arms overhead.

There are many benefits linked to working out the upper body, including improving our motor skills and preserving our range of motion. Of course, one of the best benefits of working out in the upper body is the potential for improved metabolism, which bodes well for digestion and body composition in general.

UPPER BODY EXERCISES

These exercises can easily be modified with the addition of weights or resistance bands if needed. Simple household items (like that can of soup hiding in the cupboard) can be used to add gentle weight to the workout, slowly building your stamina over time.

Chair Push-ups

- Stand tall and face a sturdy chair. Rest both hands on the back of the chair. Your feet should be a comfortable distance (roughly two steps) from the chair.

- Bend forward, hinging at the hips to keep the back straight. Make sure your core remains engaged. Keep your knees soft, with a slight bend. Gently lower yourself towards the chair, making sure that your elbows don't flare out to the sides. Go as low as you comfortably can before straightening your arms once more. Repeat as many sets and reps as needed.

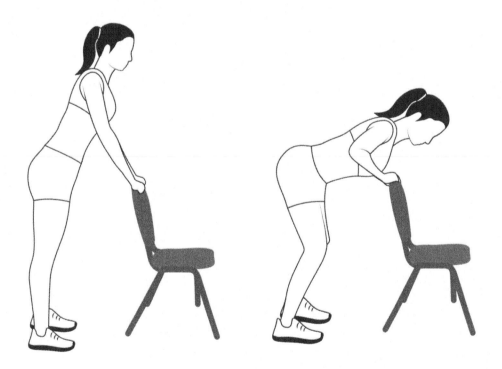

Figure 46: Chair Push-ups

Wall Push-ups

- Firmly plant your palms on the wall and take a step or two backward. Keep your back straight and the core engaged.

- Slowly lower your chest towards the wall. Be mindful to keep your elbows from splaying out to the sides. Now, straighten your arms once more.

- Complete as many sets and reps as needed.

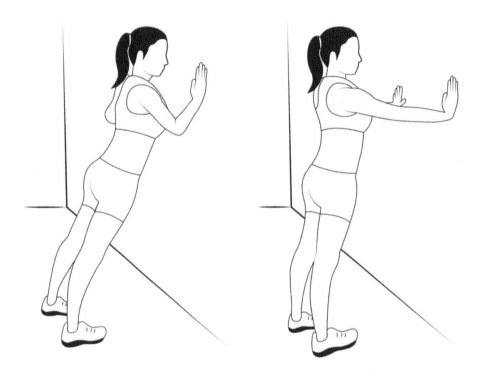

Figure 47: Wall Push-ups

Bent Over Rows

- This exercise can be done while standing or sitting. If you are standing, lean over a table or sturdy counter to assist you. If you are sitting down, simply lean over your knee. Hold a light weight in one hand and support yourself with the other.

- Inhale and lift the weight using the back of your arm until your elbow is in line with the shoulder. Exhale and slowly lower the arm to its starting position. Keep your movements slow and controlled as you continue the exercise for a set number of repetitions.

- Keep your posture straight as you complete the exercise and repeat it on the other side.

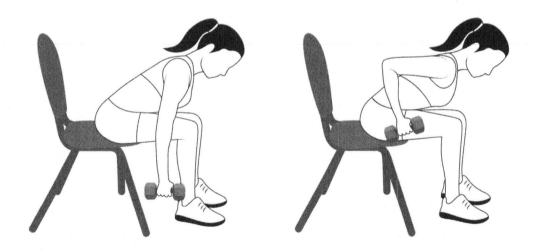

Figure 48: Bent Over Rows

Upright Rows

- Grip some light weights in both hands, keeping them at hip level. Your feet should be hip-width apart.

- Lift the weights upwards to your chin, bending the elbows. Make sure to keep the wrists straight throughout the exercise. Slowly return your hands to their starting position and repeat the exercise for the desired number of sets and reps.

- When this exercise becomes too easy, try switching to a resistance band or using slightly heavier weights.

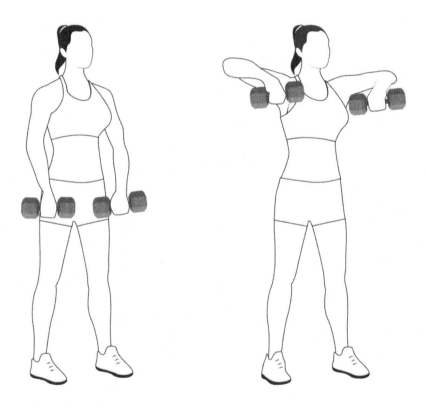

Figure 49: Upright Rows

Shoulder Rolls

- Stand tall and grip light weights in your hands. Keep your arms relaxed at your side with your feet shoulder-width apart.

- Inhale and raise your shoulders, bringing them close to the ears. Exhale and continue rolling the shoulders backward and down, returning them to the starting position. Repeat as many times as desired.

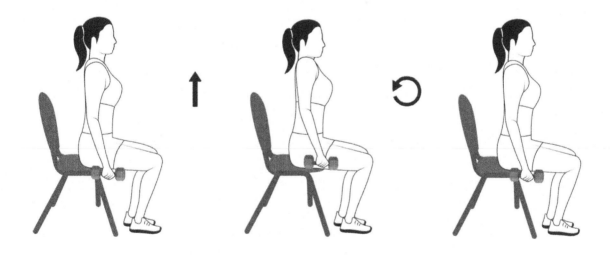

Figure 50: Shoulder Rolls

Shoulder Press-Up

- Stand with your feet shoulder-width apart. Grip a pair of weights and hold them just above the shoulders.

- Slowly raise and straighten your arms, pushing the weights above your head. Be careful not to lock your elbows. Gently return your arms to the starting position and repeat the exercise for a set number of repetitions. When you find this exercise becomes too easy, simply increase the number of repetitions or switch to a heavier weight.

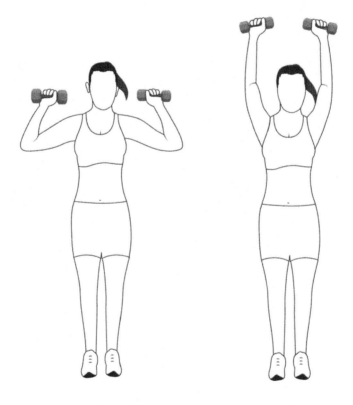

Figure 51: Shoulder Press-Up

Seated Rows

- Take a seat in a sturdy chair and hold a pair of light weights in front of your body with arms extended. Your palms should be facing each other. Try to keep the weights at a 90-degree angle.

- Slowly bring the weights closer to your body, keeping them at chest level. Squeeze your elbows behind your back to support the movement. Next, bring your arms back to their starting position and repeat the exercise several times.

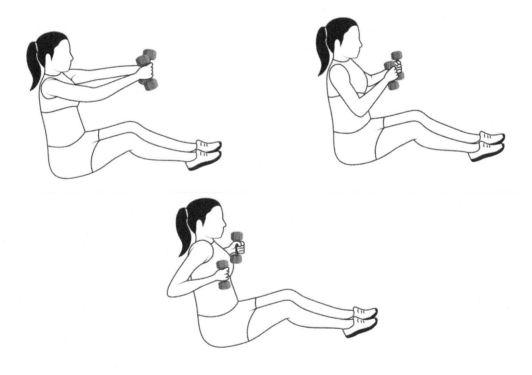

Figure 52: Seated Rows

Bicep Curls

- Stand tall, keeping your back straight and your arms by your sides. Grab a pair of weights, ensuring that your palms are facing upward. Next, curl the weights towards your shoulders and slowly lower them again. Keep your body still and your elbows close to your body to ensure that your arms are doing the actual work.

- If the exercise becomes too easy, consider switching to resistance bands or heavier weights.

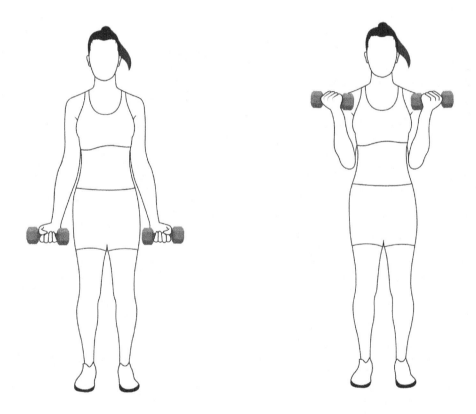

Figure 53: Bicep Curls

Tricep Kickbacks

- Stand tall with your feet comfortably apart and your knees soft. Rest your hands on your hips. Next, you'll need to hinge at the hips as you bend forward. Keep your elbows at a 90-degree angle.

- Slowly extend your forearms behind you, straightening the arms completely. Keep your arms close to your side while doing this. Return your arms to their starting position and repeat and complete the exercise with the desired number of reps.

- If balancing is difficult, work on one arm at a time and place the other on a stable surface.

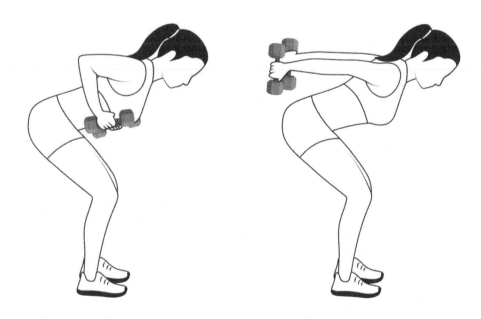

Figure 54: Tricep Kickbacks

Scapula Retractions

- Sit tall in a sturdy chair with shoulders drawn away from the ears.

- Gently place your hands on your hips, bringing the shoulders forward as you round your upper back.

- Exhale and gently drop your shoulders as you pull your elbows back to squeeze the shoulder blades. Try to keep your shoulders down throughout the exercise. Complete as many sets and reps as desired.

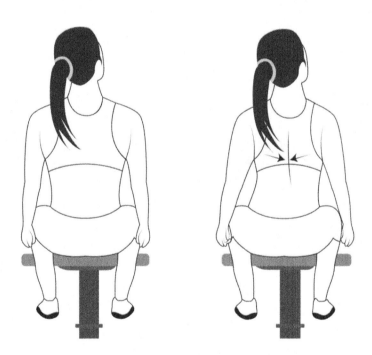

Figure 55: Scapula Retractions

Neck Side Flexions

- Sitting tall in a sturdy chair, move your head gently to the side. The goal is to bring your ear as close as you comfortably can to your shoulder. Hold the position briefly, before returning your head to an upright position. Repeat on the other side.

- Be sure not to lift your shoulders during this exercise. Otherwise, you won't feel the effects on your neck.

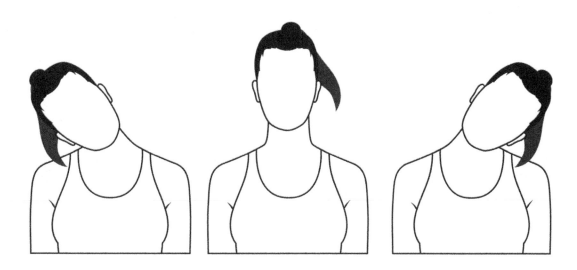

Figure 56: Neck Side Flexions

Chin Tucks

- Maintain your straight posture in the chair and slowly draw your chin back, lining the ears up with the shoulders. Slowly tuck the chin. Make sure that your head remains stationary during this movement and that you maintain your upright posture. Repeat the exercise as many times as desired.

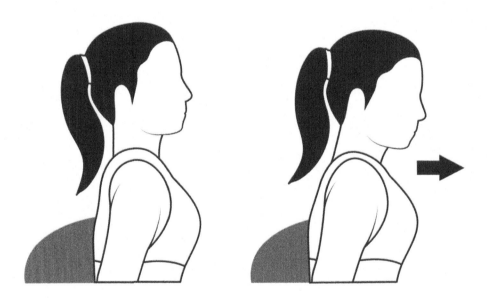

Figure 57: Chin Tucks

Side Shoulder Raise

- Stand tall, resting your arms comfortably at your sides. Grip a pair of light weights, ensuring that your palms face forward.

- Raise one arm out to the side, bringing the weight up in a wide arc. Aim to bring it over your head. In a controlled motion, bring the arm back to the starting position. Repeat as many times as desired and copy on the opposite side.

- This exercise can be made more challenging by starting with your weights in an overhead position, moving the arm in a wide arc downwards, and then returning to the overhead position. Make sure to keep your elbows straight during the exercise.

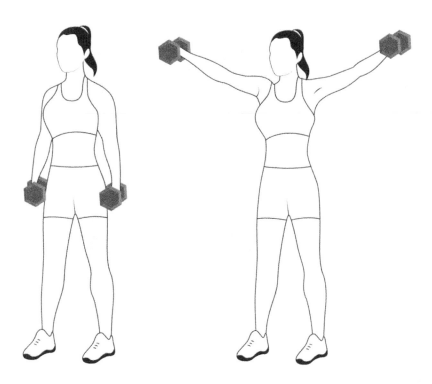

Figure 58: Side Shoulder Raises

Elbow Side Extensions

- Stand tall and strong, planting your feet shoulder-distance apart. Grip a pair of weights, bending the elbows and facing the palms towards your chest.

- Exhale as you slowly straighten your arms towards the sides. Inhale as you return your arms to their starting position and repeat. Be sure to keep your wrists straight when handling weights!

Now that we've strengthened our upper body, it is time to work on the lower body. Walking is a great way to start building lower-body strength, but the exercises in the next chapter will help you build muscle and maintain flexibility.

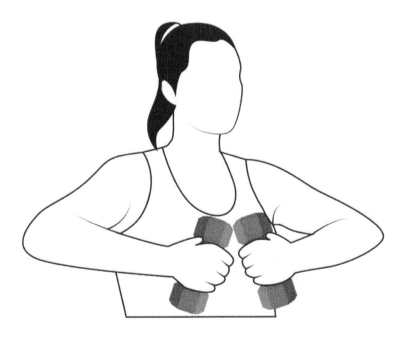

Figure 59: Elbow Side Extension - Part 1

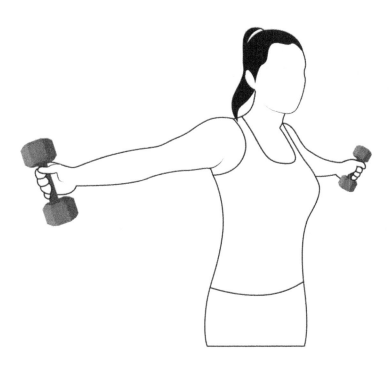

Figure 60: Elbow Side Extension - Part 2

CHAPTER 6

EXERCISES FOR THE LOWER BODY

Worries about pain, slips, and falls become increasingly common as we grow older. That is why it is beneficial to understand how we can improve our balance and strength in the lower body. Doing so will help us move with confidence and help preserve mobility. This chapter will take a look at various muscle groups in the lower body as well as exercises. Let's take a look at the muscles first.

- **Calf Muscles:** Three different muscles come together to form the calves, running from the back of the knee to the heel. These muscles help us to maintain balance and assist in walking.

- **Quadriceps:** Commonly called "quads" these muscles are located at the front of the thigh and span from the hip to the knee. Our quads are the powerhouses of the lower body and help to get up from chairs, climb stairs, walk and run.

- **Hamstrings:** Located at the back of our thighs, the hamstrings run from the buttocks to the top of the calf. These muscles help us flex and bend the knee, but they also help to stabilize the knee and play a role in dynamic activities. Tight hamstrings are a common cause of knee pain (Wilson, 2018).

- **Hip Muscles:** The muscles located in the hip are critical. They provide mobility and stability functions, enabling three-dimensional movement. These muscles also serve as a joining point between the spine and lower body, so taking care of our hip muscles is a good way to preserve mobility in our golden years.

- **Gluteal Muscles:** Our glutes support the lumbar spine and can contribute to chronic lower back pain if the muscles are weak. That's because our body is highly adaptive and will make use of other muscles to keep us moving, but this can result in potential injury and pain. So taking care of our glutes now can help us lead a pain-free life later.

- **Hip Abductors and Flexors:** These muscles are responsible to keep the pelvis level when we stand and move and contribute to overall stability and balance.

- **Hip External Rotators**: Without this group of muscles, it would be near impossible to cross our ankle over the opposite knee. Apart from moving the hip eternally, these muscles also contribute to joint stability in the hip while standing and during activities.

- **Abductors:** These are in essence our inner thigh and groin muscles, and they help to propel the leg toward the midline of our bodies and stabilize the hip joints.

EXERCISES TO STRENGTHEN THE LOWER BODY

There are a lot of muscles playing a stabilizing role in the lower body, and working out the lower body consistently will result in many positives. Improved balance and reduced pain in our hips, knees, feet, and lower back are some of the benefits we can reap. A balanced fitness program can potentially correct muscle imbalances and strengthen our bones as well, all of which are vital to remaining independent well into our golden years.

Standing and Lying Leg Exercises

These exercises help to strengthen and tone the legs, build muscle, and get rid of flabby thighs. Pay careful attention to your alignment during these exercises.

Squat

- Stand tall and plant your feet shoulder-width apart. Your toes should be pointing forward or can be turned slightly to the side. Hold on to a chair if you need help maintaining your balance.

- Now for the tricky part: Keep your core engaged and back straight as you hinge at the hips. The action is similar to sitting down in a chair. Go as low as you can manage, but try to maintain a 90-degree angle in your knees. As you rise, use both legs to propel your body upwards to straighten it. Do not use momentum to straighten yourself. Your muscles need to do the work. Your knees should not stray past your toes during this exercise.

- Complete your desired sets and reps, being mindful to keep your movements slow.

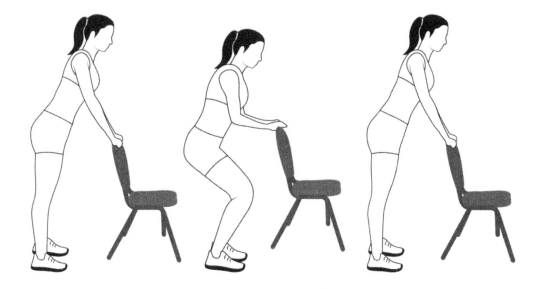

Figure 61: Squat

Partial Squat

- Stand tall and place your feet shoulder distance apart. Your toes can face outwards, slightly inwards. Grip a chair to steady yourself if needed.

- Engage your core and slowly bend at the hips as if you'll be sitting in a chair. Maintain a 45-degree angle in the knee. Use your legs to straighten your body once more. Avoid using momentum to propel yourself through this exercise. It needs to be executed slowly and thoughtfully. Be careful to keep your knees in line with your toes and that they do not stray.

- Repeat as many times as desired.

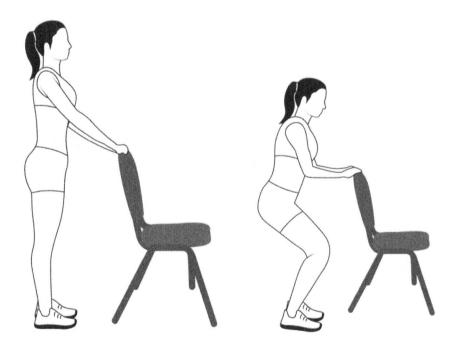

Figure 62: Partial Squat

Sit to Stand

- Sit tall and towards the front in a sturdy chair. Plant your feet at shoulder distance. Gently shift your feet backward to bring your heels behind the knees.

- Place your hands on your tights (or the armrest) and lean forward using your hips. Your nose should be over your toes now. Slowly stand up, using your legs.

- When your legs are fully extended, sit back down. Remember to bend at the hips. Keep your knees in line with your toes as you continue to repeat the exercise.

- To make this exercise more challenging, try using a lower chair or crossing your arms.

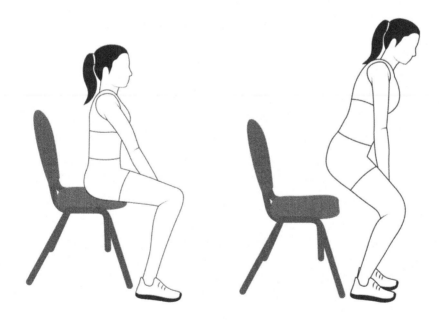

Figure 63: Sit to Stand

Reverse Lunges

- Stand tall and rest both hands on a sturdy chair. Take one step backward, lowering yourself towards the floor in the process. Go as far as you can manage.

- Use your legs to rise and repeat the exercise with the opposite leg. Your body should remain upright while you exercise, and the knee of the leading leg should not stray beyond your toes.

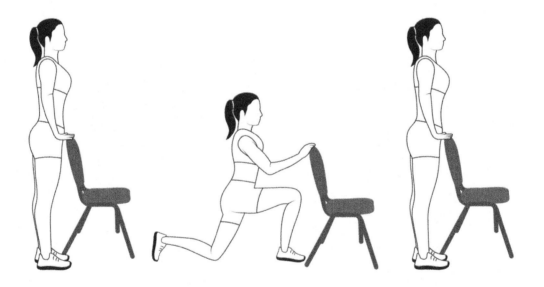

Figure 64: Reverse Lunges

Chair Deadlift

- You'll need a resistance band and chair for this exercise. Place the band flat on the floor and take a seat towards the front of a sturdy chair. Plant your feet at shoulder distance, stepping on the resistance band. Keep your knees in line with your toes.

- Next, reach down and take hold of the resistance band. With a straight back and arms, maintain your grip on the resistance band as you stand up. You'll need to completely straighten your body, squeezing your buttocks at the top of the movement. Now slowly sit down again. Repeat the exercise as many times as needed.

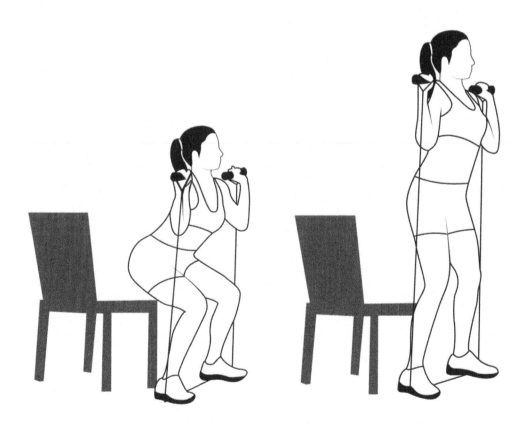

Figure 65: Chair Deadlift

Calf Raises

- Stand tall, with your feet hip distance apart. Keep your knees straight and soft as you hold onto a chair for support.

- Slowly raise yourself to your toes, lifting your heels clean off the floor. Hold the pose briefly and gently lower yourself again. Slow and steady is the key here! Don't rush as you complete the exercise.

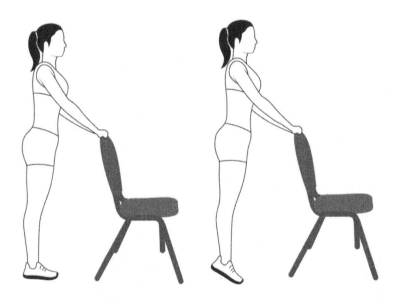

Figure 66: Calf Raises

Knee Flexions

- Stand tall, holding on to a chair. Keep your feet close together and gently bend one leg at the knee. Bring your foot as close to your buttocks as you can manage and briefly hold the position.

- Slowly return your foot to the starting position and complete the exercise. Repeat with the other leg.

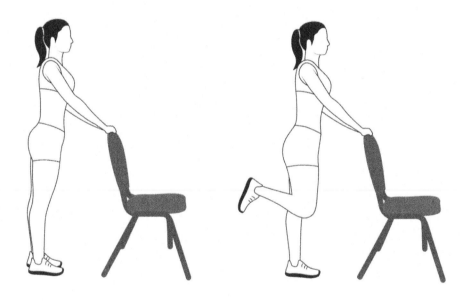

Figure 67: Knee Flexions

Hip Abductions

- Stand tall, placing your feet close together. Hold on to a chair for support.

- Now slowly raise your leg out to the side. Go as high as you can, before bringing your feet back together again. Try not to lean on the chair as you complete the exercise. Complete your desired sets and reps.

- Repeat with the other leg.

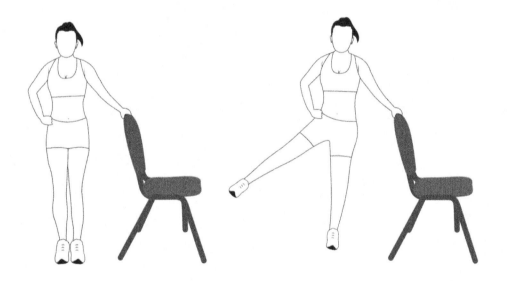

Figure 68: Hip Abductions

Hip Extensions

- Stand tall and rest your hands on a sturdy chair. Keep your legs straight and slowly move one leg behind you.

- Return your leg and plant your foot at hip distance. Repeat as many times as desired and copy with the opposite leg.

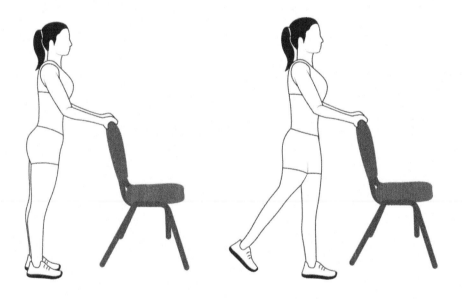

Figure 69: Hip Extensions

Hip Flexions

- Standing tall and using a chair for support, slowly lift one knee. Try to bring your thigh parallel to the floor. Hold the pose briefly and gently return your foot to the floor. Make sure that your hips remain squared throughout the exercise.

- Complete your sets and repeat on the opposite side.

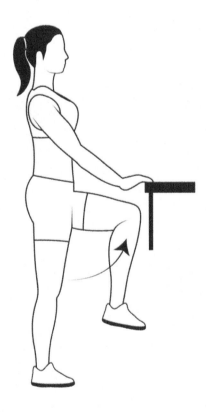

Figure 70: Hip Flexions

Lunges

- Stand tall with your hands on your hips. Your feet should be shoulder distance apart.

- Take a large step forward as you keep your trunk straight. Use your legs to push yourself up to the starting position once more. Repeat as many times as needed and switch sides. Avoid using momentum to power through this exercise. Slow and steady is the key!

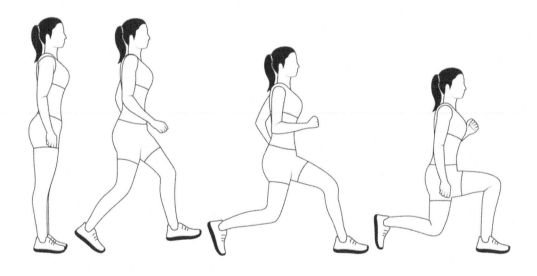

Figure 71: Lunges

Step-Ups

- A staircase or low platform can be used to do this simple exercise. Step onto the stair, bringing both feet to rest on top of it. Now step down again. Repeat as many times as desired and switch sides, leading with the other foot this time.

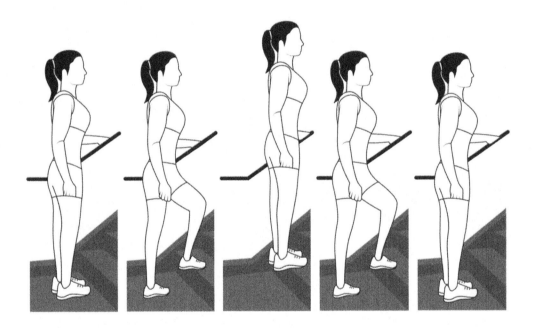

Figure 72: Step-Ups

Straight Leg Raise

- Lie comfortably on your back. Bend one knee, but keep the other straight. Keep your toes pointed to the ceiling.

- Carefully raise the straight leg, bringing it as high as your bent knee. Return your leg to the floor and repeat for your desired amount of reps. Copy with the other leg.

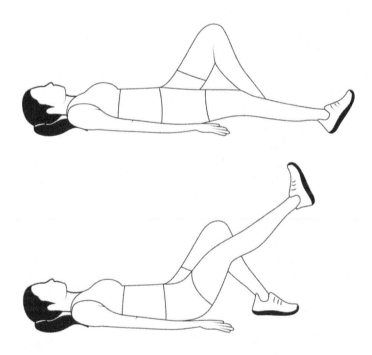

Figure 73: Straight Leg Raise

Seated Leg Exercises

The exercises in this section will add some variety to your workout routine to create balanced and strong muscles.

Seated Knee Extensions

- Sit tall and draw your shoulders down and away from the ears. Slowly raise one leg, straightening the knee to bring your foot in front of you.

- Hold the position briefly as you squeeze your quads before lowering the leg once more. Keep your movements slow and controlled as you complete your set. Repeat on the opposite side.

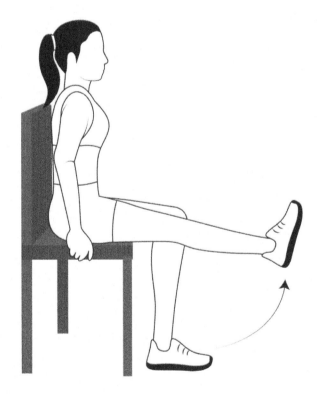

Figure 74: Seated Knee Extensions

Seated Knee Flexions

- Sit towards the front of a sturdy chair. Gently slide one foot back towards the back, going as far as you can manage.

- Return your leg to the starting position and repeat as many times as desired. Copy with the opposite leg. Keep in mind that your movements should be controlled and slow.

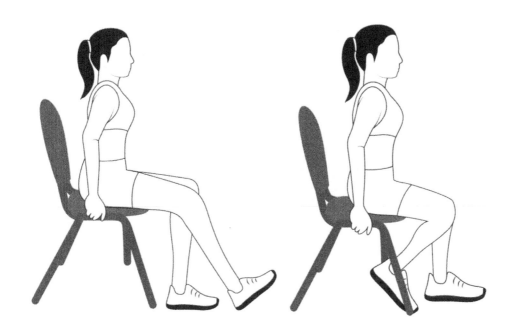

Figure 75: Seated Knee Flexions

Seated Calf Raises

- Sit tall in your chair, placing your feet hip distance apart. Slide your feet backward, bringing the heels behind the knees.

- From here, simply lift your heels from the floor. Keep your toes firmly grounded the entire time. Hold the position briefly before gently lowering the heels. Complete your desired number of sets and reps.

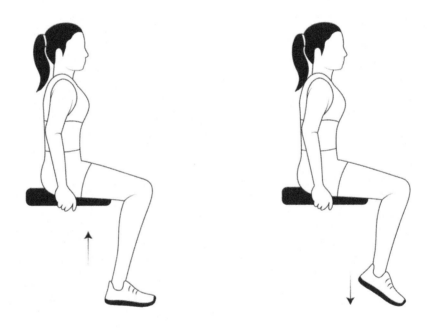

Figure 76: Seated Calf Raises

Seated Hip Flexions

- Sit tall in a sturdy chair with your shoulders drawn away from the ears.

- Slowly raise one leg, keeping the knee comfortably bent. Hold the position briefly before lowering your leg once more. Complete your set and repeat with the opposite leg.

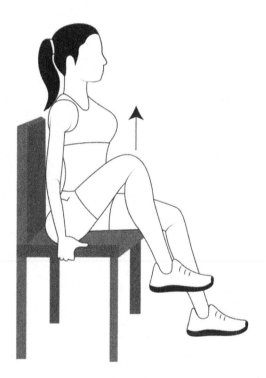

Figure 77: Seated Hip Flexions

Seated Hip Abductions

- Sit tall, with feet planted hip distance apart. Rest your hands on the outside of your knees. Now use your knees and push into your hands.

- Use your hands to apply equal pressure to the knees, resisting the force. Hold this position for several seconds, then relax. Continue to repeat the exercise until the set is complete.

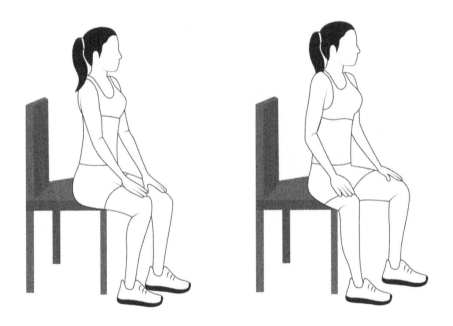

Figure 78: Seated Hip Abductions

Now that we've examined different exercises for the core, upper, and lower body, it is time to put all that knowledge to good use! In the next chapter, we'll combine these exercises into an exciting 28-day fitness program that is designed to leave you looking and feeling fantastic.

CHAPTER 7

FOUR WEEKS TO A HEALTHIER YOU

The four-week workout plan in this chapter follows a predictable pattern. Every day starts with a warm-up and some light cardio. This is followed by a targeted exercise for the arms, core, or lower body. Finally, your workout will be closed with a cool-down routine. It is recommended to start with five reps for each exercise. If this is too much (or too little), feel free to adjust the number of reps to suit your needs. You may notice that we'll refer to "sets" here and there as well. We can consider sets to be a group of repetitions. For example, if we decide on two sets of bicep curls, we'll need to perform the exercise 10 times (five repetitions per set, multiplied by two). Divide your sets however you like, and don't forget to take a small 30–60-second break between bouts of activity. Start with light weights (or no weight) and slowly work your way up to heavier weights. If you feel anything is amiss (like a pull, twinge, pain, or a feeling that something is not right), stop immediately. These workouts are fun and simple, but they can be challenging too!

DAY 1: UPPER BODY

Warm-Up

- Walking (5–10 minutes)
- Arm Opener
- Shoulder and Arm Stretch
- Standing Chest Stretch

Exercises

- Chair Push-ups: Five reps, two sets
- Wall Push-ups: Five reps, two sets
- Bent Over Rows: Five reps, two sets

Cool-Down

- Walking (5–10 minutes)
- Overhead Stretch
- Seated Chest Stretch
- Wrist Extension Stretch

DAY 2: LOWER BODY

Warm-Up

- Walking (5–10 minutes)
- Standing Hamstring Stretch
- Standing Quadricep Stretch
- Ankle Stretch

Exercises

- Seated Knee Extensions: Five reps, two sets
- Seated Knee Flexions: Five reps, two sets
- Seated Calf Raises: Five reps, two sets

Cool-Down

- Walking (5–10 minutes)
- Calf Stretch
- Lying Hamstring Stretch
- Lying Quadricep Stretch

DAY 3: CORE

Warm-Up

- Walking (5–10 minutes)
- Thoracic Extension
- Seated Hamstring Stretch
- Lumbar Extension

Exercises

- Seated Forward Roll-Ups: five reps, two sets
- Superman: Five reps, two sets
- Glute Bridges: Five reps, two sets

Cool-Down

- Walking (5–10 minutes)
- Thoracic Rotation
- Lying Hamstring Stretch
- Lumbar Flexion

DAY 4: UPPER BODY

Warm-Up

- Walking (5–10 minutes)
- Levator Scapula Stretch
- Thoracic Extension
- Rhomboids Stretch

Exercises

- Upright Rows: Five reps, two sets
- Shoulder Rolls: Five reps, two sets
- Shoulder Press-up: Five reps, two sets

Cool-Down

- Walking (5–10 minutes)
- Overhead Stretch
- Shoulder Cross-Arm Stretch
- Thoracic Rotation

DAY 5: LOWER BODY

Warm-Up

- Walking (5–10 minutes)
- Hip Abductor Stretch
- Hip Flexion Stretch
- Lying Hamstring Stretch

Exercises

- Straight Leg Raise: Five reps, two sets
- Seated Hip Flexions: Five reps, two sets
- Seated Hip Abductions: Five reps, two sets

Cool-Down

- Walking (5–10 minutes)
- Seated Hamstring Stretch
- Abductor Stretch
- Lying Hip Stretch

DAY 6: CORE

Warm-Up

- Walking (5–10 minutes)
- Thoracic Extension
- Standing Quadricep Stretch
- Lumbar Flexion

Exercises

- Seated Side Bends: Five reps, two sets
- Seated Leg Taps: Five reps, two sets
- Wood Chops: Five reps, two sets

Cool-Down

- Walking (5–10 minutes)
- Thoracic Rotation
- Lying Quadricep Stretch
- Lumbar Side Stretch

DAY 7: UPPER BODY

Warm-Up

- Walking (5–10 minutes)
- Neck Flexion Stretch
- Overhead Stretch
- Rhomboids Stretch

Exercises

- Seated Rows: Five reps, two sets
- Scapula Retractions: Five reps, two sets
- Neck Side Flexions: Five reps, two sets

Cool-Down

- Walking (5–10 minutes)
- Shoulder Cross-Arm Stretch
- Seated Chest Stretch
- Thoracic Rotation

DAY 8: LOWER BODY

Warm-Up

- Walking (5–10 minutes)
- Standing Quadricep Stretch
- Ankle Stretch
- Lumbar Extension

Exercises

- Partial Squat: Five reps, two sets
- Reverse Lunges: Five reps, two sets
- Calf Raises: Five reps, two sets

Cool-Down

- Walking (5–10 minutes)
- Calf Stretch
- Seated Hamstring Stretch
- Lying Hip Stretch

DAY 9: CORE

Warm-Up

- Walking (5–10 minutes)
- Overhead Stretch
- Hip Flexion Stretch
- Lying Hamstring Stretch

Exercises

- Seated Leg Lifts: Five reps, two sets
- Forearm Planks: Hold the pose for five seconds, and complete two sets
- Deadbug: Five reps, two sets

Cool-Down

- Walking (5–10 minutes)
- Shoulder and Arm Stretch
- Thoracic Extension
- Standing Hamstring Stretch

DAY 10: UPPER BODY

Warm-Up

- Walking (5–10 minutes)
- Levator Scapula Stretch
- Neck Side Stretch
- Overhead Stretch

Exercises

- Bicep Curls: Five reps, two sets
- Tricep Kickbacks: Five reps, two sets
- Chin Tucks: Five reps, two sets

Cool-Down

- Walking (5–10 minutes)
- Chin Drop
- Arm Opener
- Shoulder Cross-Arm Stretch

DAY 11: LOWER BODY

Warm-Up

- Walking (5–10 minutes)
- Downward Dog
- Standing Quadricep Stretch
- Lying Quadricep Stretch

Exercises

- Sit to Stand: Five reps, two sets
- Chair Deadlift: Five reps, two sets
- Knee Flexions: Five reps, two sets

Cool-Down

- Walking (5–10 minutes)
- Downward Dog
- Standing Quadricep Stretch
- Lying Quadricep Stretch

DAY 12: CORE

Warm-Up

- Walking (5–10 minutes)
- Thoracic Extension
- Seated Hamstring Stretch
- Lumbar Extension

Exercises

- Seated Forward Roll-Ups: five reps, two sets
- Superman: Five reps, two sets
- Glute Bridges: Five reps, two sets

Cool-Down

- Walking (5–10 minutes)
- Thoracic Rotation
- Lying Hamstring Stretch
- Lumbar Flexion

DAY 13: UPPER BODY

Warm-Up

- Walking (5–10 minutes)
- Neck Extension Stretch
- Shoulder and Arm Stretch
- Standing Chest Stretch

Exercises

- Chin Tucks: Five reps, two sets
- Side Shoulder Raises: Five reps, two sets
- Elbow Side Extensions: Five reps, two sets

Cool-Down

- Walking (5–10 minutes)
- Neck Rotation Stretch
- Seated Chest Stretch
- Thoracic Extension

DAY 14: LOWER BODY

Warm-Up

- Walking (5–10 minutes)
- Hip Abductor Stretch
- Standing Quadricep Stretch
- Abductor Stretch

Exercises

- Squat: Five reps, two sets
- Hip Abductions: Five reps, two sets
- Lunges: Five reps, two sets

Cool-Down

- Walking (5–10 minutes)
- Hip Flexion Stretch
- Hip Lateral Rotation Stretch
- Lying Quadricep Stretch

DAY 15: CORE

Warm-Up

- Walking (5–10 minutes)
- Thoracic Extension
- Standing Quadricep Stretch
- Lumbar Flexion

Exercises

- Seated Side Bends: Five reps, two sets
- Seated Leg Taps: Five reps, two sets
- Wood Chops: Five reps, two sets

Cool-Down

- Walking (5–10 minutes)
- Thoracic Rotation
- Lying Quadricep Stretch
- Lumbar Side Stretch

DAY 16: UPPER BODY

Warm-Up

- Walking (5–10 minutes)
- Arm Opener
- Shoulder and Arm Stretch
- Standing Chest Stretch

Exercises

- Chair Push-ups: Five reps, two sets
- Wall Push-ups: Five reps, two sets
- Bent Over Rows: Five reps, two sets

Cool-Down

- Walking (5–10 minutes)
- Overhead
- Seated Chest
- Wrist Flexion Stretch

DAY 17: LOWER BODY

Warm-Up

- Walking (5–10 minutes)
- Hip Abductor Stretch
- Hip Flexion Stretch
- Ankle Stretch

Exercises

- Seated Calf Raises: Five reps, two sets
- Seated Hip Flexions: Five reps, two sets
- Seated Hip Abductions: Five reps, two sets

Cool-Down

- Walking (5–10 minutes)
- Calf Stretch
- Hip Lateral Rotation Stretch
- Abductor Stretch

DAY 18: CORE

Warm-Up

- Walking (5–10 minutes)
- Overhead Stretch
- Hip Flexion Stretch
- Lying Hamstring Stretch

Exercises

- Seated Leg Lifts: Five reps, two sets
- Forearm Planks: Hold the pose for five seconds, and complete two sets
- Deadbug: Five reps, two sets

Cool-Down

- Walking (5–10 minutes)
- Shoulder and Arm Stretch
- Thoracic Extension
- Standing Hamstring Stretch

DAY 19: UPPER BODY

Warm-Up

- Walking (5–10 minutes)
- Levator Scapula Stretch
- Thoracic Extension
- Rhomboids Stretch

Exercises

- Upright Rows: Five reps, two sets
- Shoulder Rolls: Five reps, two sets
- Shoulder Press-up: Five reps, two sets

Cool-Down

- Walking (5–10 minutes)
- Overhead Stretch
- Shoulder Cross-Arm Stretch
- Thoracic Rotation

DAY 20: LOWER BODY

Warm-Up

- Walking (5–10 minutes)
- Standing Hamstring Stretch
- Standing Quadricep Stretch
- Hip Flexion Stretch

Exercises

- Hip Extensions: Five reps, two sets
- Hip Flexions: Five reps, two sets
- Step-Ups: Five reps, two sets

Cool-Down

- Walking (5–10 minutes)
- Lying Hamstring Stretch
- Lying Quadricep Stretch
- Lying Hip Stretch

DAY 21: CORE

Warm-Up

- Walking (5–10 minutes)
- Thoracic Extension
- Seated Hamstring Stretch
- Lumbar Extension

Exercises

- Seated Forward Roll-Ups: five reps, two sets
- Superman: Five reps, two sets
- Glute Bridges: Five reps, two sets

Cool-Down

- Walking (5–10 minutes)
- Thoracic Rotation
- Lying Hamstring Stretch
- Lumbar Flexion

DAY 22: UPPER BODY

Warm-Up

- Walking (5–10 minutes)
- Neck Flexion Stretch
- Overhead Stretch
- Rhomboids Stretch

Exercises

- Seated Rows: Five reps, two sets
- Scapula Retractions: Five reps, two sets
- Neck Side Flexions: Five reps, two sets

Cool-Down

- Walking (5–10 minutes)
- Shoulder Cross-Arm Stretch
- Seated Chest Stretch
- Thoracic Rotation

DAY 23: LOWER BODY

Warm-Up

- Walking (5–10 minutes)
- Seated Hamstring Stretch
- Ankle Stretch
- Lumbar Flexion

Exercises

- Squat: Five reps, two sets
- Reverse Lunges: Five reps, two sets
- Calf Raises: Five reps, two sets

Cool-Down

- Walking (5–10 minutes)
- Downward Dog
- Calf Stretch
- Lumbar Extension

DAY 24: CORE

Warm-Up

- Walking (5–10 minutes)
- Thoracic Extension
- Standing Quadricep Stretch
- Lumbar Flexion

Exercises

- Seated Side Bends: Five reps, two sets
- Seated Leg Taps: Five reps, two sets
- Wood Chops: Five reps, two sets

Cool-Down

- Walking (5–10 minutes)
- Thoracic Rotation
- Lying Quadricep Stretch
- Lumbar Side Stretch

DAY 25: UPPER BODY

Warm-Up

- Walking (5–10 minutes)
- Levator Scapula Stretch
- Neck Side Stretch
- Overhead Stretch

Exercises

- Bicep Curls: Five reps, two sets
- Tricep Kickbacks: Five reps, two sets
- Chin Tucks: Five reps, two sets

Cool-Down

- Walking (5–10 minutes)
- Chin Drop
- Arm Opener
- Shoulder Cross-Arm Stretch

DAY 26: LOWER BODY

Warm-Up

- Walking (5–10 minutes)
- Standing Quadricep Stretch
- Lying Quadricep Stretch
- Lumbar Flexion

Exercises

- Sit to Stand: Five reps, two sets
- Chair Deadlift: Five reps, two sets
- Knee Flexions: Five reps, two sets

Cool-Down

- Walking (5–10 minutes)
- Downward Dog
- Calf Stretch
- Lumbar Extension

DAY 27: CORE

Warm-Up

- Walking (5–10 minutes)
- Overhead Stretch
- Hip Flexion Stretch
- Lying Hamstring Stretch

Exercises

- Seated Leg Lifts: Five reps, two sets
- Forearm Planks: Hold the pose for five seconds, and complete two sets
- Deadbug: Five reps, two sets

Cool-Down

- Walking (5–10 minutes)
- Shoulder and Arm Stretch
- Thoracic Extension
- Standing Hamstring Stretch

DAY 28: UPPER BODY

Warm-Up

- Walking (5–10 minutes)
- Neck Extension Stretch
- Shoulder and Arm Stretch
- Standing Chest Stretch

Exercises

- Chin Tucks: Five reps, two sets
- Side Shoulder Raises: Five reps, two sets
- Elbow Side Extensions: Five reps, two sets

Cool-Down

- Walking (5–10 minutes)
- Neck Rotation Stretch
- Seated Chest Stretch
- Thoracic Extension

This 28-day program is a great introduction to your fitness journey! You can repeat the exercises as many times as you like. As you continue your fitness journey, feel free to experiment with your breaks, weights, and number of repetitions to push yourself closer to your goals.

CONCLUSION

Now that you have all the information you need, it is time to kick-start your fitness journey. You can conquer pain, regain your mobility, and achieve those fitness goals you've been putting off. After reading this book, you should feel confident in your knowledge about warm-ups, stretches, and cool-downs and how important they are too a balanced fitness program.

Remember, even people who have health conditions and other physical considerations are still able to remain physically active. Just consult your health practitioner first before attempting a fitness routine, as there may be some exercises that should be avoided. Just like Chivonne, whose story I shared at the start of the book, you too can live an active life well into your golden years. Don't spend another minute doubting yourself or feeling weak. You have the power to take your life back!

If you enjoyed this book, please consider leaving a review. It will be an inspiring pleasure to hear how far you've come in your fitness journey!

REFERENCES

10 drug-free ways to control high blood pressure. (n.d.). Mayo Clinic. https://www.mayoclinic.org/diseases-conditions/high-blood-pressure/in-depth/high-blood-pressure/art-20046974#:~:text=For%20those%20who%20have%20hypertension

Abdominal muscles. (2012). Better Health Channel. https://www.betterhealth.vic.gov.au/health/conditionsandtreatments/abdominal-muscles

Angulo, J., El Assar, M., Álvarez-Bustos, A., & Rodríguez-Mañas, L. (2020). Physical activity and exercise: Strategies to manage frailty. *Redox Biology*, 35, 101513. https://doi.org/10.1016/j.redox.2020.101513

Benefits of Increasing Upper Body Strength. (2021, April 15). Integrated Rehabilitation Services. https://integrehab.com/blog/strength-and-conditioning/upper-body-strength/#:~:text=A%20strong%20upper%20body%20can

Bilodeau, K. (2019, March 8). *Stretching: Less pain, other gains.* Harvard Health Blog. https://www.health.harvard.edu/blog/stretching-less-pain-other-gains-2019030816168

Blaszczak, J. (2016, May 17). *Get in the Right Mindset to Exercise Regularly.* Psych Central. https://psychcentral.com/lib/get-in-the-right-mindset-to-exercise-regularly#1

Carter, S. (2022, June 15). *Why are core muscles important?* Livescience. https://www.livescience.com/why-are-core-muscles-important

Colberg, S. R., Sigal, R. J., Yardley, J. E., Riddell, M. C., Dunstan, D. W., Dempsey, P. C., Horton, E. S., Castorino, K., & Tate, D. F. (2016). Physical Activity/Exercise and Diabetes: a Position Statement of the American Diabetes Association. *Diabetes Care*, 39(11), 2065–2079. https://doi.org/10.2337/dc16-1728

Core Muscles. (n.d.). Physiopedia. https://www.physio-pedia.com/Core_Muscles

Cristopoliski, F., Barela, J. A., Leite, N., Fowler, N. E., & Rodacki, A. L. F. (2009). *Stretching Exercise Program Improves Gait in the Elderly.* Gerontology, 55(6), 614–620. https://doi.org/10.1159/000235863

Deltoid Muscles: What Are They, Anatomy, Location & Function. (2021). Cleveland Clinic. https://my.clevelandclinic.org/health/body/21875-deltoid-muscles#:~:text=Your%20deltoid%20muscles%20are%20in

Edwards, T., & Ward, S. (2022, February 15). *How to Engage Your Core: Steps, Muscles Worked, and More.* Healthline. https://www.healthline.com/nutrition/how-to-engage-your-core#:~:text=Transversus%20abdominis&text=It

Endorphins: The brain's natural pain reliever. (2021, July 20). Harvard Health Publishing. https://www.health.harvard.edu/mind-and-mood/endorphins-the-brains-natural-pain-reliever#:~:text=You%20can%20increase%20your%20body

Exercise for Chronic Pain Management - 7 Tips. (2022, March 14). CORA Physical Therapy. https://www.coraphysicaltherapy.com/exercise-for-chronic-pain-management/

Exercise: Rx for overcoming osteoarthritis. (2019, June 24). Harvard Health. https://www.health.harvard.edu/staying-healthy/exercise-rx-for-overcoming-osteoarthritis

Exercises to help prevent falls. (2020). Medlineplus. https://medlineplus.gov/ency/patientinstructions/000493.htm#:~:text=Exercising%20can%20help%20prevent%20falls

Galloway, J. (2022, May 23). *3 Signs of Weak Glutes a PT Says to Watch Out For.* Well+Good. https://www.wellandgood.com/signs-weak-glutes/

Gopez, J. (2017, October 11). *Stretching for Back Pain Relief.* Spine-Health. https://www.spine-health.com/wellness/exercise/stretching-back-pain-relief

Iliades, MD, C. (2018, April 30). *What Counts as Aerobic Exercise (aka Cardio).* EverydayHealth. https://www.everydayhealth.com/fitness/workouts/why-you-need-aerobic-exercise.aspx

Importance of Stretching. (n.d.). Orthopedic and Sports Medicine Institute (OSMI). https://www.osmifw.com/the-importance-of-stretching/

Jeno, S. H., & Varacallo, M. (2021). *Anatomy, Back, Latissimus Dorsi. PubMed; StatPearls* Publishing. https://www.ncbi.nlm.nih.gov/books/NBK448120/#:~:text=The%20latissimus%20dorsi%20muscle%20is

Kuehn, K. (2021, July 8). *40 Body Positive Quotes Everyone Should Read.* Reader's Digest. https://www.rd.com/article/body-positive-quotes/

Langhammer, B., Bergland, A., & Rydwik, E. (2018). The Importance of Physical Activity Exercise among Older People. *BioMed Research International*, 2018(1), 1–3. https://doi.org/10.1155/2018/7856823

Livingston, G., Sommerlad, A., Orgeta, V., Costafreda, S. G., Huntley, J., Ames, D., Ballard, C., Banerjee, S., Burns, A., Cohen-Mansfield, J., Cooper, C., Fox, N., Gitlin, L. N., Howard, R., Kales, H. C., Larson, E. B., Ritchie, K., Rockwood, K., Sampson, E. L., & Samus, Q. (2017). Dementia prevention, intervention, and care. *The Lancet,* 390(10113), 2673–2734. https://doi.org/10.1016/s0140-6736(17)31363-6

Maintaining mobility and preventing disability are key to living independently as we age. (2020, November 30). National Institute on Aging. https://www.nia.nih.gov/news/maintaining-mobility-and-preventing-disability-are-key-living-independently-we-age

Move More; Sit Less. (2022, March 17). Centers for Disease Control and Prevention. https://www.cdc.gov/physicalactivity/basics/adults/index.htm#:~:text=Each%20week%20adults%20need%20150

Physical Activity and the Person with Cancer. (2022, March 16). American Cancer Society. https://www.cancer.org/treatment/survivorship-during-and-after-treatment/be-healthy-after-treatment/physical-activity-and-the-cancer-patient.html#:~:text=Research%20shows%20that%20for%20most

Physical activity for seniors. (2012). Better Health Channel. https://www.betterhealth.vic.gov.au/health/healthyliving/physical-activity-for-seniors

Physical inactivity a leading cause of disease and disability, warns WHO. (2002, April 4). WHO. https://www.who.int/news/item/04-04-2002-physical-inactivity-a-leading-cause-of-disease-and-disability-warns-who

Roser, M., Ortiz-Ospina, E., & Ritchie, H. (2013). *Life Expectancy*. Our World in Data. https://ourworldindata.org/life-expectancy#:~:text=Globally%20the%20life%20expectancy%20increased

Sherrington, C., Tiedemann, A., & Cameron, I. (2011). Physical exercise after hip fracture: an evidence overview. *European Journal of Physical and Rehabilitation Medicine, 47*(2), 297–307. https://pubmed.ncbi.nlm.nih.gov/21555983/#:~:text=Physical%20exercise%20has%20the%20potential

Stelter, G. (2014, August 14). *5 Seated Back Pain Stretches for Seniors*. Healthline. https://www.healthline.com/health/back-pain/stretches-for-seniors

Thieme, T. (2021, January 25). *Your Core Muscles Are More Than Just Abs*. Men's Health. https://www.menshealth.com/fitness/a35307843/core-muscles/

Volpi, E., Nazemi, R., & Fujita, S. (2004). Muscle tissue changes with aging. *Current Opinion in Clinical Nutrition and Metabolic Care, 7*(4), 405–410. https://www.ncbi.nlm.nih.gov/pmc/articles/PMC2804956/#:~:text=Muscle%20mass%20decreases%20approximately%203

Watson, S. (2020, November 23). *Balance Training: Benefits, Intensity Level, and More*. WebMD. https://www.webmd.com/fitness-exercise/a-z/balance-training#:~:text=Examples%20of%20balance%20exercises%20include

Why Warming Up and Cooling Down is Important. (2016, December 15). Tri-City Medical Center. https://www.tricitymed.org/2016/12/warming-cooling-important/

Wilson, C. (2018, September 28). *Hamstring Stretches To Relieve Pain & Tightness*. Wilson Health. https://www.knee-pain-explained.com/hamstring-stretches.html

Ylinen, J., Wirén, K., & Häkkinen, A. (2007). Stretching exercises vs manual therapy in treatment of chronic neck pain: a randomized, controlled cross-over trial. *Journal of Rehabilitation Medicine, 39*(2), 126–132. https://doi.org/10.2340/16501977-001